BRUXISM

A MEDICAL DICTIONARY, BIBLIOGRAPHY,
AND ANNOTATED RESEARCH GUIDE TO
INTERNET REFERENCES

JAMES N. PARKER, M.D.
AND PHILIP M. PARKER, PH.D., EDITORS

ii

ICON Health Publications
ICON Group International, Inc.
4370 La Jolla Village Drive, 4th Floor
San Diego, CA 92122 USA

Printed in the United States of America.

Last digit indicates print number: 10 9 8 7 6 4 5 3 2 1

Publisher, Health Care: Philip Parker, Ph.D.
Editor(s): James Parker, M.D., Philip Parker, Ph.D.

Publisher's note: The ideas, procedures, and suggestions contained in this book are not intended for the diagnosis or treatment of a health problem. As new medical or scientific information becomes available from academic and clinical research, recommended treatments and drug therapies may undergo changes. The authors, editors, and publisher have attempted to make the information in this book up to date and accurate in accord with accepted standards at the time of publication. The authors, editors, and publisher are not responsible for errors or omissions or for consequences from application of the book, and make no warranty, expressed or implied, in regard to the contents of this book. Any practice described in this book should be applied by the reader in accordance with professional standards of care used in regard to the unique circumstances that may apply in each situation. The reader is advised to always check product information (package inserts) for changes and new information regarding dosage and contraindications before prescribing any drug or pharmacological product. Caution is especially urged when using new or infrequently ordered drugs, herbal remedies, vitamins and supplements, alternative therapies, complementary therapies and medicines, and integrative medical treatments.

Cataloging-in-Publication Data

Parker, James N., 1961-
Parker, Philip M., 1960-

Bruxism: A Medical Dictionary, Bibliography, and Annotated Research Guide to Internet References / James N. Parker and Philip M. Parker, editors
        p.   cm.
Includes bibliographical references, glossary, and index.
ISBN: 0-497-00187-X
1. Bruxism-Popular works.   I. Title.

Disclaimer

This publication is not intended to be used for the diagnosis or treatment of a health problem. It is sold with the understanding that the publisher, editors, and authors are not engaging in the rendering of medical, psychological, financial, legal, or other professional services.

References to any entity, product, service, or source of information that may be contained in this publication should not be considered an endorsement, either direct or implied, by the publisher, editors, or authors. ICON Group International, Inc., the editors, and the authors are not responsible for the content of any Web pages or publications referenced in this publication.

Copyright Notice

Acknowledgements

The collective knowledge generated from academic and applied research summarized in various references has been critical in the creation of this book which is best viewed as a comprehensive compilation and collection of information prepared by various official agencies which produce publications on bruxism. Books in this series draw from various agencies and institutions associated with the United States Department of Health and Human Services, and in particular, the Office of the Secretary of Health and Human Services (OS), the Administration for Children and Families (ACF), the Administration on Aging (AOA), the Agency for Healthcare Research and Quality (AHRQ), the Agency for Toxic Substances and Disease Registry (ATSDR), the Centers for Disease Control and Prevention (CDC), the Food and Drug Administration (FDA), the Healthcare Financing Administration (HCFA), the Health Resources and Services Administration (HRSA), the Indian Health Service (IHS), the institutions of the National Institutes of Health (NIH), the Program Support Center (PSC), and the Substance Abuse and Mental Health Services Administration (SAMHSA). In addition to these sources, information gathered from the National Library of Medicine, the United States Patent Office, the European Union, and their related organizations has been invaluable in the creation of this book. Some of the work represented was financially supported by the Research and Development Committee at INSEAD. This support is gratefully acknowledged. Finally, special thanks are owed to Tiffany Freeman for her excellent editorial support.

About the Editors

James N. Parker, M.D.

Dr. James N. Parker received his Bachelor of Science degree in Psychobiology from the University of California, Riverside and his M.D. from the University of California, San Diego. In addition to authoring numerous research publications, he has lectured at various academic institutions. Dr. Parker is the medical editor for health books by ICON Health Publications.

Philip M. Parker, Ph.D.

Philip M. Parker is the Eli Lilly Chair Professor of Innovation, Business and Society at INSEAD (Fontainebleau, France and Singapore). Dr. Parker has also been Professor at the University of California, San Diego and has taught courses at Harvard University, the Hong Kong University of Science and Technology, the Massachusetts Institute of Technology, Stanford University, and UCLA. Dr. Parker is the associate editor for ICON Health Publications.

About ICON Health Publications

To discover more about ICON Health Publications, simply check with your preferred online booksellers, including Barnes&Noble.com and Amazon.com which currently carry all of our titles. Or, feel free to contact us directly for bulk purchases or institutional discounts:

ICON Group International, Inc.
4370 La Jolla Village Drive, Fourth Floor
San Diego, CA 92122 USA
Fax: 858-546-4341
Web site: **www.icongrouponline.com/health**

Table of Contents

FORWARD

In March 2001, the National Institutes of Health issued the following warning: "The number of Web sites offering health-related resources grows every day. Many sites provide valuable information, while others may have information that is unreliable or misleading."[1] Furthermore, because of the rapid increase in Internet-based information, many hours can be wasted searching, selecting, and printing. Since only the smallest fraction of information dealing with bruxism is indexed in search engines, such as **www.google.com** or others, a non-systematic approach to Internet research can be not only time consuming, but also incomplete. This book was created for medical professionals, students, and members of the general public who want to know as much as possible about bruxism, using the most advanced research tools available and spending the least amount of time doing so.

In addition to offering a structured and comprehensive bibliography, the pages that follow will tell you where and how to find reliable information covering virtually all topics related to bruxism, from the essentials to the most advanced areas of research. Public, academic, government, and peer-reviewed research studies are emphasized. Various abstracts are reproduced to give you some of the latest official information available to date on bruxism. Abundant guidance is given on how to obtain free-of-charge primary research results via the Internet. **While this book focuses on the field of medicine, when some sources provide access to non-medical information relating to bruxism, these are noted in the text.**

E-book and electronic versions of this book are fully interactive with each of the Internet sites mentioned (clicking on a hyperlink automatically opens your browser to the site indicated). If you are using the hard copy version of this book, you can access a cited Web site by typing the provided Web address directly into your Internet browser. You may find it useful to refer to synonyms or related terms when accessing these Internet databases. **NOTE:** At the time of publication, the Web addresses were functional. However, some links may fail due to URL address changes, which is a common occurrence on the Internet.

For readers unfamiliar with the Internet, detailed instructions are offered on how to access electronic resources. For readers unfamiliar with medical terminology, a comprehensive glossary is provided. For readers without access to Internet resources, a directory of medical libraries, that have or can locate references cited here, is given. We hope these resources will prove useful to the widest possible audience seeking information on bruxism.

The Editors

---

[1] From the NIH, National Cancer Institute (NCI): **http://www.cancer.gov/cancerinfo/ten-things-to-know**.

Chapter 1. Studies on Bruxism

Overview

In this chapter, we will show you how to locate peer-reviewed references and studies on bruxism.

The Combined Health Information Database

The Combined Health Information Database summarizes studies across numerous federal agencies. To limit your investigation to research studies and bruxism, you will need to use the advanced search options. First, go to **http://chid.nih.gov/index.html**. From there, select the "Detailed Search" option (or go directly to that page with the following hyperlink: **http://chid.nih.gov/detail/detail.html**). The trick in extracting studies is found in the drop boxes at the bottom of the search page where "You may refine your search by." Select the dates and language you prefer, and the format option "Journal Article." At the top of the search form, select the number of records you would like to see (we recommend 100) and check the box to display "whole records." We recommend that you type "bruxism" (or synonyms) into the "For these words:" box. Consider using the option "anywhere in record" to make your search as broad as possible. If you want to limit the search to only a particular field, such as the title of the journal, then select this option in the "Search in these fields" drop box. The following is what you can expect from this type of search:

- **Treating Severe Bruxism with Botulinum Toxin**

  Source: JADA. Journal of the American Dental Association. 131(2): 211-216. February 2000.

  Contact: Available from American Dental Association. ADA Publishing Co, Inc., 211 East Chicago Avenue, Chicago, IL 60611.

  Summary: Locally administered botulinum toxin (BTX) is an effective treatment for various movement disorders. This article reports on a study that investigated the use of BTX as a treatment for severe **bruxism** (tooth grinding). The authors studied 18 subjects with severe **bruxism** and whose mean duration of symptoms was 14.8 years (range of three to 40 years). These subjects audibly ground their teeth and experienced tooth wear and difficulty speaking, swallowing, or chewing. Medical or dental procedures had failed to alleviate their symptoms. The authors administered a total of 241 injections of BTX type A in the subjects' masseter muscles during 123 treatment visits. The mean total duration of response was 19.1 weeks (range of six to 78 weeks), and the mean peak effect on a scale of 0 to 4, in which 4 is equal to total abolishment of grinding, was 3.4. Only one subject (5.6 percent) reported having experienced dysphagia was BTX A. The results of this study suggest that BTX administered by skilled practitioners is a safe and effective treatment for people with severe **bruxism,** particularly those with associated movement disorders. However, BTX treatment should be considered only for those patients refractory to conventional therapy. 2 tables. 33 references.

- **Effect of Bruxism on Treatment Planning for Dental Implants**

Source: Dentistry Today. 21(9): 76-78, 80-81. September 2002.

Contact: Available from Dentistry Today Inc. 26 Park Street, Montclair, NJ 07042. (973) 783-3935.

Summary: There is general agreement that excessive stress to the bone-implant interface in dental implants may result in implant overload and failure. This article considers the role of **bruxism** (grinding of the teeth) on treatment planning for dental implants. Topics include stress and force, normal bite force, parafunction, **bruxism,** diagnosis, implant fatigue fractures, occlusal guards, implant design, and fracture. The author reiterates that **bruxism** is a potential risk factor for implant failure. Excessive force is the primary cause of late implant complications. Once the dentist has identified the source(s) of additional force on the implant system, the treatment plan is altered to contend with and reduce the negative sequelae on the bone, implant, and final restoration. For example, additional implants can be placed to decrease stress on any one implant, and implants in molar regions should have an increased width. Night guards designed with specific features also are a benefit to initially diagnose the influence of occlusal factors for the patient, and as importantly, to reduce the influence of extraneous stress on implants and implant-retained restorations. Appended to the article is a posttest for continuing education credits. 10 figures. 23 references.

- **Treating Bruxism and Clenching**

Source: JADA. Journal of the American Dental Association. 131(2): 233-235. February 2000.

Contact: Available from American Dental Association. ADA Publishing Co, Inc., 211 East Chicago Avenue, Chicago, IL 60611.

Summary: This article discusses several concepts to aid dental practitioners in the treatment of patients with **bruxism (tooth grinding)** or clenching of the jaws. The author first reviews the problems of **bruxism** and clenching, then discusses treatment of the young patient (during the mixed dentition period) with **bruxism** or clenching, the use of occlusal splints, nighttime and daytime use of the splints, treatment of the middle aged patient with **bruxism** or clenching, restorative treatment, and rehabilitation issues. The author cautions that **bruxism** or clenching can cause total destruction of the dentition if allowed to progress without patient education or preventive therapy. Conversely, proper patient education as soon as **bruxism** or clenching is observed, acceptable restoration of affected teeth and wearing of an acrylic resin splint allow the patient with **bruxism** or clenching to live a normal life, without significant tooth wear or other dental handicaps. 1 reference.

- **Effect of a Full-Arch Maxillary Occlusal Splint on Parafunctional Activity During Sleep in Patients With Nocturnal Bruxism and Signs and Symptoms of Craniomandibular Disorders**

  Source: Journal of Prosthetic Dentistry. 69(3): 293-297. March 1993.

  Summary: This article reports on a study to investigate the effects of the occlusal splint on parafunctional oral motor behavior (grinding and clenching) during sleep in patients with **bruxism** and craniomandibular disorders. The results revealed that the splint does not stop nocturnal **bruxism**. In 61 percent of the patients, wear facets on the splint were observed at every visit (2-week intervals) and in 39 percent, from time to time. The wear facets reappeared in the same location with the same pattern and were caused mainly by grinding. The extension of the facets showed that during eccentric **bruxism,** the mandible moved laterally far beyond the edge-to-edge contact relationship of the canines. 5 figures. 15 references. (AA).

Federally Funded Research on Bruxism

The U.S. Government supports a variety of research studies relating to bruxism. These studies are tracked by the Office of Extramural Research at the National Institutes of Health.[2] CRISP (Computerized Retrieval of Information on Scientific Projects) is a searchable database of federally funded biomedical research projects conducted at universities, hospitals, and other institutions.

Search the CRISP Web site at **http://crisp.cit.nih.gov/crisp/crisp_query.generate_screen**. You will have the option to perform targeted searches by various criteria, including geography, date, and topics related to bruxism.

For most of the studies, the agencies reporting into CRISP provide summaries or abstracts. As opposed to clinical trial research using patients, many federally funded studies use animals or simulated models to explore bruxism. The following is typical of the type of information found when searching the CRISP database for bruxism:

- **Project Title: BRAINSTEM MECHANISMS CONTROLLING JAW MOVEMENTS**

  Principal Investigator & Institution: Chandler, Scott H.; Inst for Social Sci Research; University of California Los Angeles 10920 Wilshire Blvd., Suite 1200 Los Angeles, Ca 90024

  Timing: Fiscal Year 2003; Project Start 01-AUG-1983; Project End 31-MAR-2008

  Summary: (provided by applicant): The proper functioning of oral-facial motor systems is necessary for the survival of humans. The ingestive behaviors of mammals begins with suckling and progresses to drinking and chewing. Presently, there are very few studies addressing how the brain is organized to produce these behaviors. Even less is known about the etiology of various oral-motor disorders such as tardive dyskinesia, **bruxism,** and myofacial pain dysfunction syndromes. The long-term goals of this research are to understand both the mechanisms underlying the central nervous system control of normal jaw movements that occur during activities such as drinking and

---

[2] Healthcare projects are funded by the National Institutes of Health (NIH), Substance Abuse and Mental Health Services (SAMHSA), Health Resources and Services Administration (HRSA), Food and Drug Administration (FDA), Centers for Disease Control and Prevention (CDCP), Agency for Healthcare Research and Quality (AHRQ), and Office of Assistant Secretary of Health (OASH).

chewing, as well as the abnormal jaw movements that occur during various disorders. The specific aims of this proposal are to continue investigations, at the cellular level, into the neuronal mechanisms controlling trigeminal neuronal membrane excitability and burst discharge that are associated with the critical transition from primitive suckling behavior to adult-like mastication in the rat. We will combine whole cell patch clamp recording methods of neurons within the trigeminal nuclei responsible for oral-motor activity (mesencephalic V neurons and trigeminal interneurons) in brain slices with microstimulation, neurochemical, and mathematical modeling techniques to more fully elucidate 1) the mechanisms controlling excitability, and 2) the local chemical and electrical microcircuitry of these neurons. The project is divided into two Specific Aims. In Specific Aim I we will determine the locations of, and ionic mechanisms underlying, intrinsic burst generation in Mes V and trigeminal interneurons in the vicinity of the trigeminal motor nucleus and test the hypothesis that the underlying conductances are substrates for modulation by metabotropic glutamate receptor (mGluR) and serotonergic (5-HT) receptor activation. Specific Aim II focuses on characterizing the local excitatory and inhibitory chemical and electrical synaptic interactions that occur between distinct trigeminal neurons, and the modulation of these interactions by activation of mGluR and 5-HT receptors. The results of the proposed studies will provide insights into the local microcircuitry and the cellular mechanisms controlling discharge of distinct populations of trigeminal neurons involved in production of jaw movements at distinct developmental time points, and will serve as a cellular foundation for creation of neuronal models of masticatory rhythm and burst pattern generation.

Website: http://crisp.cit.nih.gov/crisp/Crisp_Query.Generate_Screen

- **Project Title: CONTROL OF AIRWAY MOTOR NEURONS DURING SLEEP/WAKEFULNESS**

Principal Investigator & Institution: Siegel, Jerome M.; Professor; Brain Research Institute; University of California Los Angeles 10920 Wilshire Blvd., Suite 1200 Los Angeles, Ca 90024

Timing: Fiscal Year 2002; Project Start 01-SEP-1998; Project End 31-AUG-2003

Summary: The loss of upper airway muscle tone in sleep is the precipitating cause of sleep apnea. Sleep apnea affects 3-5% of men over 40 and 1.5-2.5% of post-menopausal women. It causes persistent sleepiness, exacerbates a variety of medical conditions and increases morbidity and mortality. We will study how forebrain sleep induction mechanisms cause the reduction of muscle tone in airway dilators. A variety of complementary techniques will be used in sleep apnea patients to determine which forebrain and brainstem regions are activated and inactivated during airway obstruction. In projects 2 and 3 the pathways from forebrain sleep inducing regions will be traced to the brainstem region activated and inactivated in sleep apnea, focusing on regions controlling upper airway muscle tone. These studies will use anatomical tract tracing techniques, thermal activation of sleep controlling neurons and unit recording in the posterior hypothalamus, periaqueductal gray and medulla of unrestrained animals. In projects 4 and 5 we will determine which amino acid and monoamine transmitters mediate the suppression of muscle tone in airway dilator motoneurons during REM and non-REM sleep. These studies will use in vivo microdialysis, intracellular unit recording and iontophoresis. This program will bring basic science techniques to bear on the important clinical problem of sleep apnea. Pilot studies for this collaborative enterprise have already yield data that will produce a major revision in our understanding of the mechanisms controlling the airway during sleep. The work of this SCOR (Specialized

Center of Research) will increase our understanding of sleep apnea. It is also likely to be of importance to other disorders of motor control during sleep. It is also likely to be of importance to other disorders of motor control during sleep, including REM sleep behavior disorder, **bruxism,** periodic limb movements during sleep and cataplexy. This research will also shed light on the cellular mechanisms controlling REM and non-REM sleep states.

Website: http://crisp.cit.nih.gov/crisp/Crisp_Query.Generate_Screen

- **Project Title: PARAFUNCTIONAL ACTIVITY AND TEMPOROMANDIBULAR DISORDERS**

  Principal Investigator & Institution: Glaros, Alan G.; Beulah Mccullom Professor; Dental Public Health & Behav Scis; University of Missouri Kansas City Kansas City, Mo 64110

  Timing: Fiscal Year 2002; Project Start 15-SEP-2000; Project End 30-JUN-2004

  Summary: (adapted from the investigator's abstract): Temporomandibular disorders (TMD) are a heterogeneous collection of disorders characterized by orofacial pain and/or masticatory dysfunction. Parafunctional behaviors, especially clenching and grinding, are presumed to be important initiating and perpetuating factors in TMD (Glaros & Glass, 1993). Recent studies have showed that low-level parafunctional activity in otherwise normal individuals increases pain and can produce the same symptoms of TMD reported by clinic patients. However, there is very little direct evidence that TMD patients engage in more parafunctional activities than others or that the parafunctional activities that they may engage in are related to pain. The specific aims of this project are therefore to test the hypotheses that (1) TMD patients engage in higher rates of parafunctional activities than a comparable non-TMD sample, and (2) parafunctional activities produce and/or increase pain. Both in vivo and laboratory-based studies will be conducted to test the hypotheses. One of the proposed studies will utilize a methodologically sophisticated, ecologically valid self-report technique known as ecological momentary assessment (EMA). EMA data are a sample of the participant's behavior, emotional state, or physiological states in the real world, and these data can be examined for co-variation among the variables in time. The long-term objectives of this research are: (1) to better describe and characterize some basic, essential differences among TMD and non-TMD subjects; (2) to develop an etiological theory of TMD which adequately accounts for the observed differences; and (3) to develop effective treatment programs for TMD derived from our improved understanding of this disorder.

  Website: http://crisp.cit.nih.gov/crisp/Crisp_Query.Generate_Screen

- **Project Title: THE ROLE OF TOOTH MECHANORECEPTORS IN JAW MOVEMENT**

  Principal Investigator & Institution: Dessem, Dean A.; Associate Professor; Oral & Craniofacial Biol Scis; University of Maryland Balt Prof School Baltimore, Md 21201

  Timing: Fiscal Year 2002; Project Start 01-JUL-1991; Project End 31-AUG-2007

  Summary: (provided by applicant): The long-term objectives of this project are to determine the role of craniofacial sensory feedback in normal function and to determine how these processes are altered in oro-facial dysfunctions including **bruxism,** masticatory muscle and temporomandibular disorders. Three hypotheses are proposed: 1) Trigeminal ganglion jaw muscle and joint primary afferent neurons comprise two general categories with brainstem axonal projections correlated to their functional modalities. Hypothesis 1 will be tested by characterizing the physiological and morphological properties of these neurons using in vivo intracellular recording and staining. 2) Sensory feedback from non-spindle muscle and joint afferents is relayed directly to trigeminothalamic, trigeminohypothalamic, trigemino-parabrachial, trigeminospinal and trigeminal premotor neurons. These pathways are expected to convey discriminative, autonomic and emotional aspects of orofacial nociception; as well as innocuous proprioceptive and autonomic sensory feedback. Hypothesis 2 will be tested by characterizing neuronal circuitry from trigeminal ganglion muscle and joint afferents to brainstem neurons by combining in vivo retrograde and intracellular neuronal labeling. 3) Transmission from trigeminal ganglion neurons relaying feedback from muscle and joint to brainstem neurons can be modulated via presynaptic mechanisms. It is also predicted that primary afferent depolarization (PAD) and centrifugal action potentials can be evoked in these afferent axons which may induce neurogenic inflammation. Hypothesis 3 will be tested by determining if the anatomical substrate for presynaptic modulation of non-spindle muscle and jaw joint afferent terminals is present using intracellular labeling, confocal and electron microscopy. This hypothesis will also be tested by directly monitoring the membrane potential in primary afferent axons using in vivo intra-axonal recording during electrical and chemical stimulation of orofacial tissues. Mechanisms of PAD will be explored using GABAA and GABAB agonists and antagonists. Data from experiments in this proposal will provide better understanding of the morphology and physiology of deep orofacial primary afferent neurons and their brainstem circuitry. This knowledge will not only lead to a better understanding of brain mechanisms but is needed to develop rational treatment strategies for managing musculoskeletal and orofacial disorders. These data will also be used to investigate potential gender differences in the morphological substrate and physiological mechanisms of primary afferent neurons involved in musculoskeletal and orofacial disorders including musculoskeletal pain, temporomandibular disorders (TMD), fibromyalgia and myofacial pain.

Website: http://crisp.cit.nih.gov/crisp/Crisp_Query.Generate_Screen

The National Library of Medicine: PubMed

One of the quickest and most comprehensive ways to find academic studies in both English and other languages is to use PubMed, maintained by the National Library of Medicine.[3] The advantage of PubMed over previously mentioned sources is that it covers a greater number of domestic and foreign references. It is also free to use. If the publisher has a Web site that offers full text of its journals, PubMed will provide links to that site, as well as to sites offering other related data. User registration, a subscription fee, or some other type of fee may be required to access the full text of articles in some journals.

To generate your own bibliography of studies dealing with bruxism, simply go to the PubMed Web site at **http://www.ncbi.nlm.nih.gov/pubmed**. Type "bruxism" (or synonyms) into the search box, and click "Go." The following is the type of output you can expect from PubMed for bruxism (hyperlinks lead to article summaries):

---

[3] PubMed was developed by the National Center for Biotechnology Information (NCBI) at the National Library of Medicine (NLM) at the National Institutes of Health (NIH). The PubMed database was developed in conjunction with publishers of biomedical literature as a search tool for accessing literature citations and linking to full-text journal articles at Web sites of participating publishers. Publishers that participate in PubMed supply NLM with their citations electronically prior to or at the time of publication.

- A bibliographical survey of bruxism with special emphasis on non-traditional treatment modalities.
Author(s): Nissani M.
Source: J Oral Sci. 2001 June; 43(2): 73-83. Review.
http://www.ncbi.nlm.nih.gov/entrez/query.fcgi?cmd=Retrieve&db=pubmed&dopt=Abstract&list_uids=11515601

- A clinical and electromyographic study of the long-term effects of an occlusal splint on the temporal and masseter muscles in patients with functional disorders and nocturnal bruxism.
Author(s): Sheikholeslam A, Holmgren K, Riise C.
Source: Journal of Oral Rehabilitation. 1986 March; 13(2): 137-45.
http://www.ncbi.nlm.nih.gov/entrez/query.fcgi?cmd=Retrieve&db=pubmed&dopt=Abstract&list_uids=3457133

- A clinical diagnosis of diurnal (non-sleep) bruxism in denture wearers.
Author(s): Piquero K, Sakurai K.
Source: Journal of Oral Rehabilitation. 2000 June; 27(6): 473-82.
http://www.ncbi.nlm.nih.gov/entrez/query.fcgi?cmd=Retrieve&db=pubmed&dopt=Abstract&list_uids=10888274

- A factor analytic study of psychosocial background in bruxism.
Author(s): Olkinuora M.
Source: Proc Finn Dent Soc. 1972; 68(4): 184-99. No Abstract Available.
http://www.ncbi.nlm.nih.gov/entrez/query.fcgi?cmd=Retrieve&db=pubmed&dopt=Abstract&list_uids=4509012

- A modified bruxism appliance.
Author(s): Ordene NM.
Source: The New York State Dental Journal. 1989 January; 55(1): 40-1.
http://www.ncbi.nlm.nih.gov/entrez/query.fcgi?cmd=Retrieve&db=pubmed&dopt=Abstract&list_uids=2913538

- A multidimensional approach to bruxism and TMD.
Author(s): Cannistraci AJ, Friedrich JA.
Source: The New York State Dental Journal. 1987 October; 53(8): 31-4.
http://www.ncbi.nlm.nih.gov/entrez/query.fcgi?cmd=Retrieve&db=pubmed&dopt=Abstract&list_uids=3477733

- A new approach to the treatment of bruxism and bruxomania.
Author(s): Ackerman JB.
Source: The New York State Dental Journal. 1966 June-July; 32(6): 259-61.
http://www.ncbi.nlm.nih.gov/entrez/query.fcgi?cmd=Retrieve&db=pubmed&dopt=Abstract&list_uids=5220855

- A new method for recording mandibular position during nocturnal bruxism.
Author(s): Akamatsu Y, Minagi S, Sato T.
Source: Journal of Oral Rehabilitation. 1996 September; 23(9): 622-6.
http://www.ncbi.nlm.nih.gov/entrez/query.fcgi?cmd=Retrieve&db=pubmed&dopt=Abstract&list_uids=8890063

- **A new occlusal splint for treating bruxism and TMD during orthodontic therapy.**
  Author(s): Sullivan TC.
  Source: J Clin Orthod. 2001 March; 35(3): 142-4. No Abstract Available.
  http://www.ncbi.nlm.nih.gov/entrez/query.fcgi?cmd=Retrieve&db=pubmed&dopt=Abstract&list_uids=11314592

- **A piezoelectric film-based intrasplint detection method for bruxism.**
  Author(s): Takeuchi H, Ikeda T, Clark GT.
  Source: The Journal of Prosthetic Dentistry. 2001 August; 86(2): 195-202.
  http://www.ncbi.nlm.nih.gov/entrez/query.fcgi?cmd=Retrieve&db=pubmed&dopt=Abstract&list_uids=11514809

- **A procedure for making a bruxism device in the office.**
  Author(s): Austin D, Attanasio R.
  Source: The Journal of Prosthetic Dentistry. 1991 August; 66(2): 266-9.
  http://www.ncbi.nlm.nih.gov/entrez/query.fcgi?cmd=Retrieve&db=pubmed&dopt=Abstract&list_uids=1774690

- **A psycho-odontological investigation of patients with bruxism.**
  Author(s): Molin C, Levi L.
  Source: Acta Odontologica Scandinavica. 1966 November; 24(3): 373-91.
  http://www.ncbi.nlm.nih.gov/entrez/query.fcgi?cmd=Retrieve&db=pubmed&dopt=Abstract&list_uids=5225454

- **A psychosomatic study of bruxism with emphasis on mental strain and familiar predisposition factors.**
  Author(s): Olkinuora M.
  Source: Proc Finn Dent Soc. 1972; 68(3): 110-23. No Abstract Available.
  http://www.ncbi.nlm.nih.gov/entrez/query.fcgi?cmd=Retrieve&db=pubmed&dopt=Abstract&list_uids=4509076

- **A randomized double-blind clinical trial of the effect of amitriptyline on nocturnal masseteric motor activity (sleep bruxism).**
  Author(s): Mohamed SE, Christensen LV, Penchas J.
  Source: Cranio. 1997 October; 15(4): 326-32.
  http://www.ncbi.nlm.nih.gov/entrez/query.fcgi?cmd=Retrieve&db=pubmed&dopt=Abstract&list_uids=9481995

- **A review of psychogenic aspects and treatment of bruxism.**
  Author(s): Mikami DB.
  Source: The Journal of Prosthetic Dentistry. 1977 April; 37(4): 411-9.
  http://www.ncbi.nlm.nih.gov/entrez/query.fcgi?cmd=Retrieve&db=pubmed&dopt=Abstract&list_uids=191598

- **A review of the literature on the causes, effect and therapy of bruxism.**
  Author(s): James RM.
  Source: Bull Mich Dent Hyg Assoc. 1982 September; 12(3): 11-3. No Abstract Available.
  http://www.ncbi.nlm.nih.gov/entrez/query.fcgi?cmd=Retrieve&db=pubmed&dopt=Abstract&list_uids=6958341

- **A treatment for damaged anterior teeth associated with bruxism.**
  Author(s): Cosgrove DJ.
  Source: Aust Dent J. 1974 October; 19(5): 320-1. No Abstract Available.
  http://www.ncbi.nlm.nih.gov/entrez/query.fcgi?cmd=Retrieve&db=pubmed&dopt=Abstract&list_uids=4614772

- **A vibratory stimulation-based inhibition system for nocturnal bruxism: a clinical report.**
  Author(s): Watanabe T, Baba K, Yamagata K, Ohyama T, Clark GT.
  Source: The Journal of Prosthetic Dentistry. 2001 March; 85(3): 233-5.
  http://www.ncbi.nlm.nih.gov/entrez/query.fcgi?cmd=Retrieve&db=pubmed&dopt=Abstract&list_uids=11264929

- **Acute temporomandibular arthritis in a patient with bruxism and calcium pyrophosphate deposition disease.**
  Author(s): Good AE, Upton LG.
  Source: Arthritis and Rheumatism. 1982 March; 25(3): 353-5.
  http://www.ncbi.nlm.nih.gov/entrez/query.fcgi?cmd=Retrieve&db=pubmed&dopt=Abstract&list_uids=6279120

- **Alcohol and bruxism.**
  Author(s): Hartmann E.
  Source: The New England Journal of Medicine. 1979 August 9; 301(6): 333-4.
  http://www.ncbi.nlm.nih.gov/entrez/query.fcgi?cmd=Retrieve&db=pubmed&dopt=Abstract&list_uids=450031

- **Altered control of submaximal bite force during bruxism in humans.**
  Author(s): Mantyvaara J, Sjoholm T, Kirjavainen T, Waltimo A, Iivonen M, Kemppainen P, Pertovaara A.
  Source: European Journal of Applied Physiology and Occupational Physiology. 1999 March; 79(4): 325-30.
  http://www.ncbi.nlm.nih.gov/entrez/query.fcgi?cmd=Retrieve&db=pubmed&dopt=Abstract&list_uids=10090631

- **Alternative view of the bruxism phenomenon.**
  Author(s): Kreisburg MK.
  Source: Gen Dent. 1982 March-April; 30(2): 121-3. Review. No Abstract Available.
  http://www.ncbi.nlm.nih.gov/entrez/query.fcgi?cmd=Retrieve&db=pubmed&dopt=Abstract&list_uids=6749593

- **An assessment of the structure of perception in people with bruxism.**
  Author(s): Godlewski C, Pietruska MD, Stokowska W, Pietruski JK, Roslan D.
  Source: Rocz Akad Med Bialymst. 1999; 44: 47-54.
  http://www.ncbi.nlm.nih.gov/entrez/query.fcgi?cmd=Retrieve&db=pubmed&dopt=Abstract&list_uids=10697419

- **An overview of bruxism and its management.**
  Author(s): Attanasio R.
  Source: Dent Clin North Am. 1997 April; 41(2): 229-41. Review.
  http://www.ncbi.nlm.nih.gov/entrez/query.fcgi?cmd=Retrieve&db=pubmed&dopt=Abstract&list_uids=9142481

- **Antidepressant-induced bruxism successfully treated with gabapentin.**
  Author(s): Brown ES, Hong SC.
  Source: The Journal of the American Dental Association. 1999 October; 130(10): 1467-9.
  http://www.ncbi.nlm.nih.gov/entrez/query.fcgi?cmd=Retrieve&db=pubmed&dopt=Abstract&list_uids=10570590

- **Apparatus for recording of bruxism during sleep.**
  Author(s): Gentz R.
  Source: Sven Tandlak Tidskr. 1972 June; 65(6): 327-42. No Abstract Available.
  http://www.ncbi.nlm.nih.gov/entrez/query.fcgi?cmd=Retrieve&db=pubmed&dopt=Abstract&list_uids=4517201

- **Arousability and bruxism in male and female college students.**
  Author(s): Westrup DA, Keller SR, Nellis TA, Hicks RA.
  Source: Percept Mot Skills. 1992 December; 75(3 Pt 1): 796-8.
  http://www.ncbi.nlm.nih.gov/entrez/query.fcgi?cmd=Retrieve&db=pubmed&dopt=Abstract&list_uids=1454478

- **Association between nocturnal bruxism and gastroesophageal reflux.**
  Author(s): Miyawaki S, Tanimoto Y, Araki Y, Katayama A, Fujii A, Takano-Yamamoto T.
  Source: Sleep. 2003 November 1; 26(7): 888-92.
  http://www.ncbi.nlm.nih.gov/entrez/query.fcgi?cmd=Retrieve&db=pubmed&dopt=Abstract&list_uids=14655925

- **Association between sleep bruxism, swallowing-related laryngeal movement, and sleep positions.**
  Author(s): Miyawaki S, Lavigne GJ, Pierre M, Guitard F, Montplaisir JY, Kato T.
  Source: Sleep. 2003 June 15; 26(4): 461-5.
  http://www.ncbi.nlm.nih.gov/entrez/query.fcgi?cmd=Retrieve&db=pubmed&dopt=Abstract&list_uids=12841373

- **Atypical granuloma associated with compulsive bruxism in an adolescent female.**
  Author(s): Ulrich GH, Griffin JW.
  Source: J Periodontol. 1967 November-December; 38(6): 514-7. No Abstract Available.
  http://www.ncbi.nlm.nih.gov/entrez/query.fcgi?cmd=Retrieve&db=pubmed&dopt=Abstract&list_uids=5234639

- **Aversive control of bruxism in a mentally retarded child: a case study.**
  Author(s): Kramer JJ.
  Source: Psychological Reports. 1981 December; 49(3): 815-8.
  http://www.ncbi.nlm.nih.gov/entrez/query.fcgi?cmd=Retrieve&db=pubmed&dopt=Abstract&list_uids=7330146

- **Behavioral history: relationship to treatment and frequency in psychogenic bruxism.**
  Author(s): Keith KD.
  Source: J Nebr Dent Assoc. 1978 Spring; 54(3): 14-6. No Abstract Available.
  http://www.ncbi.nlm.nih.gov/entrez/query.fcgi?cmd=Retrieve&db=pubmed&dopt=Abstract&list_uids=288869

- **Bite force in children with bruxism.**
  Author(s): Lindqvist B, Rinqvist M.
  Source: Acta Odontologica Scandinavica. 1973 October; 31(4): 255-9.
  http://www.ncbi.nlm.nih.gov/entrez/query.fcgi?cmd=Retrieve&db=pubmed&dopt=Abstract&list_uids=4519511

- **Bruxism after brain injury: successful treatment with botulinum toxin-A.**
  Author(s): Ivanhoe CB, Lai JM, Francisco GE.
  Source: Archives of Physical Medicine and Rehabilitation. 1997 November; 78(11): 1272-3.
  http://www.ncbi.nlm.nih.gov/entrez/query.fcgi?cmd=Retrieve&db=pubmed&dopt=Abstract&list_uids=9365360

- **Bruxism and bruxomania.**
  Author(s): Shatkin AJ.
  Source: R I Dent J. 1992 Winter; 25(4): 7-10. No Abstract Available.
  http://www.ncbi.nlm.nih.gov/entrez/query.fcgi?cmd=Retrieve&db=pubmed&dopt=Abstract&list_uids=1306911

- **Bruxism and cold sensitivity.**
  Author(s): Wilson TG.
  Source: Quintessence Int. 2002 September; 33(8): 559. No Abstract Available.
  http://www.ncbi.nlm.nih.gov/entrez/query.fcgi?cmd=Retrieve&db=pubmed&dopt=Abstract&list_uids=12238685

- **Bruxism and cranial-cervical dystonia: is there a relationship?**
  Author(s): Watts MW, Tan EK, Jankovic J.
  Source: Cranio. 1999 July; 17(3): 196-201.
  http://www.ncbi.nlm.nih.gov/entrez/query.fcgi?cmd=Retrieve&db=pubmed&dopt=Abstract&list_uids=10650407

- **Bruxism and emotional disturbance.**
  Author(s): Lindqvist B.
  Source: Odontol Revy. 1972; 23(2): 231-42. No Abstract Available.
  http://www.ncbi.nlm.nih.gov/entrez/query.fcgi?cmd=Retrieve&db=pubmed&dopt=Abstract&list_uids=4504497

- **Bruxism and intraoral orthotics.**
  Author(s): Attanasio R.
  Source: Tex Dent J. 2000 July; 117(7): 82-7. Review. No Abstract Available.
  http://www.ncbi.nlm.nih.gov/entrez/query.fcgi?cmd=Retrieve&db=pubmed&dopt=Abstract&list_uids=11858068

- **Bruxism and its associated oral sequela in the mentally retarded patient.**
  Author(s): Greenwald MM.
  Source: J Conn State Dent Assoc. 1991 Spring; 67(1): 33-6. No Abstract Available.
  http://www.ncbi.nlm.nih.gov/entrez/query.fcgi?cmd=Retrieve&db=pubmed&dopt=Abstract&list_uids=1830322

- **Bruxism and its effect on the natural teeth.**
  Author(s): Drago CJ.
  Source: The Journal of Prosthetic Dentistry. 1986 February; 55(2): 281.
  http://www.ncbi.nlm.nih.gov/entrez/query.fcgi?cmd=Retrieve&db=pubmed&dopt=Abstract&list_uids=3457159

- **Bruxism and its effect on the natural teeth.**
  Author(s): Pavone BW.
  Source: The Journal of Prosthetic Dentistry. 1985 May; 53(5): 692-6.
  http://www.ncbi.nlm.nih.gov/entrez/query.fcgi?cmd=Retrieve&db=pubmed&dopt=Abstract&list_uids=3858535

- **Bruxism and its effect on the teeth.**
  Author(s): Xhonga FA.
  Source: Journal of Oral Rehabilitation. 1977 January; 4(1): 65-76.
  http://www.ncbi.nlm.nih.gov/entrez/query.fcgi?cmd=Retrieve&db=pubmed&dopt=Abstract&list_uids=265365

- **Bruxism and magnesium. Literature review and case reports.**
  Author(s): Lehvila P.
  Source: Proc Finn Dent Soc. 1974 December; 70(6): 217-24. No Abstract Available.
  http://www.ncbi.nlm.nih.gov/entrez/query.fcgi?cmd=Retrieve&db=pubmed&dopt=Abstract&list_uids=4457918

- **Bruxism and orofacial movements during sleep.**
  Author(s): Kato T, Thie NM, Montplaisir JY, Lavigne GJ.
  Source: Dent Clin North Am. 2001 October; 45(4): 657-84. Review.
  http://www.ncbi.nlm.nih.gov/entrez/query.fcgi?cmd=Retrieve&db=pubmed&dopt=Abstract&list_uids=11699235

- **Bruxism and periodontal disease: a critical review.**
  Author(s): Love R, Clark G.
  Source: J West Soc Periodontol Periodontal Abstr. 1978; 26(4): 104-11. Review. No Abstract Available.
  http://www.ncbi.nlm.nih.gov/entrez/query.fcgi?cmd=Retrieve&db=pubmed&dopt=Abstract&list_uids=161617

- **Bruxism and psychobiological model of personality.**
  Author(s): Jorgic-Srdjak K, Ivezic S, Cekic-Arambasin A, Bosnjak A.
  Source: Coll Antropol. 1998 December; 22 Suppl: 205-12.
  http://www.ncbi.nlm.nih.gov/entrez/query.fcgi?cmd=Retrieve&db=pubmed&dopt=Abstract&list_uids=9951165

- **Bruxism and sexual abuse.**
  Author(s): Goldman MJ, Gutheil TG.
  Source: The American Journal of Psychiatry. 1991 August; 148(8): 1089.
  http://www.ncbi.nlm.nih.gov/entrez/query.fcgi?cmd=Retrieve&db=pubmed&dopt=Abstract&list_uids=1853965

- **Bruxism and sexual abuse: a possible association?**
  Author(s): Goldman MJ, Gutheil TG.
  Source: The Journal of the American Dental Association. 1991 March; 122(3): 22.
  http://www.ncbi.nlm.nih.gov/entrez/query.fcgi?cmd=Retrieve&db=pubmed&dopt=Abstract&list_uids=2019685

- **Bruxism and the bite.**
  Author(s): Wessberg G.
  Source: Hawaii Dent J. 2001 March-April; 32(2): 4. No Abstract Available.
  http://www.ncbi.nlm.nih.gov/entrez/query.fcgi?cmd=Retrieve&db=pubmed&dopt=Abstract&list_uids=11494476

- **Bruxism and the occlusion.**
  Author(s): Arnold M.
  Source: Dent Clin North Am. 1981 July; 25(3): 395-407. No Abstract Available.
  http://www.ncbi.nlm.nih.gov/entrez/query.fcgi?cmd=Retrieve&db=pubmed&dopt=Abstract&list_uids=6943102

- **Bruxism as presenting feature of Parkinson's disease.**
  Author(s): Srivastava T, Ahuja M, Srivastava M, Trivedi A.
  Source: J Assoc Physicians India. 2002 March; 50: 457. No Abstract Available.
  http://www.ncbi.nlm.nih.gov/entrez/query.fcgi?cmd=Retrieve&db=pubmed&dopt=Abstract&list_uids=11922248

- **Bruxism following cerebellar hemorrhage.**
  Author(s): Pollack IA, Cwik V.
  Source: Neurology. 1989 September; 39(9): 1262.
  http://www.ncbi.nlm.nih.gov/entrez/query.fcgi?cmd=Retrieve&db=pubmed&dopt=Abstract&list_uids=2771078

- **Bruxism force detection by a piezoelectric film-based recording device in sleeping humans.**
  Author(s): Baba K, Clark GT, Watanabe T, Ohyama T.
  Source: J Orofac Pain. 2003 Winter; 17(1): 58-64.
  http://www.ncbi.nlm.nih.gov/entrez/query.fcgi?cmd=Retrieve&db=pubmed&dopt=Abstract&list_uids=12756932

- **Bruxism in allergic children.**
  Author(s): Marks MB.
  Source: Am J Orthod. 1980 January; 77(1): 48-59.
  http://www.ncbi.nlm.nih.gov/entrez/query.fcgi?cmd=Retrieve&db=pubmed&dopt=Abstract&list_uids=6928084

- **Bruxism in children with brain damage.**
  Author(s): Lindqvist B, Heijbel J.
  Source: Acta Odontologica Scandinavica. 1974; 32(5): 313-9.
  http://www.ncbi.nlm.nih.gov/entrez/query.fcgi?cmd=Retrieve&db=pubmed&dopt=A
  bstract&list_uids=4281989

- **Bruxism in children.**
  Author(s): Ahmad R.
  Source: J Pedod. 1986 Winter; 10(2): 105-26. No Abstract Available.
  http://www.ncbi.nlm.nih.gov/entrez/query.fcgi?cmd=Retrieve&db=pubmed&dopt=A
  bstract&list_uids=3458897

- **Bruxism in children: review of the literature.**
  Author(s): Cash RC.
  Source: J Pedod. 1988 Winter; 12(2): 107-27. Review. No Abstract Available.
  http://www.ncbi.nlm.nih.gov/entrez/query.fcgi?cmd=Retrieve&db=pubmed&dopt=A
  bstract&list_uids=3280778

- **Bruxism in Huntington's disease.**
  Author(s): Louis ED, Tampone E.
  Source: Movement Disorders : Official Journal of the Movement Disorder Society. 2001
  July; 16(4): 785-6.
  http://www.ncbi.nlm.nih.gov/entrez/query.fcgi?cmd=Retrieve&db=pubmed&dopt=A
  bstract&list_uids=11481718

- **Bruxism in Huntington's disease.**
  Author(s): Tan EK, Jankovic J, Ondo W.
  Source: Movement Disorders : Official Journal of the Movement Disorder Society. 2000
  January; 15(1): 171-3.
  http://www.ncbi.nlm.nih.gov/entrez/query.fcgi?cmd=Retrieve&db=pubmed&dopt=A
  bstract&list_uids=10634263

- **Bruxism in maxillary overdenture patients.**
  Author(s): Kirk GA.
  Source: The Journal of Prosthetic Dentistry. 1984 November; 52(5): 764.
  http://www.ncbi.nlm.nih.gov/entrez/query.fcgi?cmd=Retrieve&db=pubmed&dopt=A
  bstract&list_uids=6387104

- **Bruxism in Rett syndrome: a case report.**
  Author(s): Alpoz AR, Ergul N, Oncag O, Ergul N.
  Source: J Clin Pediatr Dent. 1999 Winter; 23(2): 161-3. Erratum In: Journal of Clinical
  Pediatric Dentistry 1999 Summer; 23(4): Following 373. Ergul N[corrected to Oncag O].
  http://www.ncbi.nlm.nih.gov/entrez/query.fcgi?cmd=Retrieve&db=pubmed&dopt=A
  bstract&list_uids=10204460

- **Bruxism in twins.**
  Author(s): Lindqvist B.
  Source: Acta Odontologica Scandinavica. 1974; 32(3): 177-87.
  http://www.ncbi.nlm.nih.gov/entrez/query.fcgi?cmd=Retrieve&db=pubmed&dopt=A
  bstract&list_uids=4613102

- **Bruxism is mainly regulated centrally, not peripherally.**
  Author(s): Lobbezoo F, Naeije M.
  Source: Journal of Oral Rehabilitation. 2001 December; 28(12): 1085-91. Review.
  http://www.ncbi.nlm.nih.gov/entrez/query.fcgi?cmd=Retrieve&db=pubmed&dopt=Abstract&list_uids=11874505

- **Bruxism levels and daily behaviors: 3 weeks of measurement and correlation.**
  Author(s): Watanabe T, Ichikawa K, Clark GT.
  Source: J Orofac Pain. 2003 Winter; 17(1): 65-73.
  http://www.ncbi.nlm.nih.gov/entrez/query.fcgi?cmd=Retrieve&db=pubmed&dopt=Abstract&list_uids=12756933

- **Bruxism masquerading as a murmur.**
  Author(s): Marinella MA.
  Source: Archives of Internal Medicine. 2002 March 11; 162(5): 606.
  http://www.ncbi.nlm.nih.gov/entrez/query.fcgi?cmd=Retrieve&db=pubmed&dopt=Abstract&list_uids=11871931

- **Bruxism secondary to antipsychotic drug exposure: a positive response to propranolol.**
  Author(s): Amir I, Hermesh H, Gavish A.
  Source: Clinical Neuropharmacology. 1997 February; 20(1): 86-9.
  http://www.ncbi.nlm.nih.gov/entrez/query.fcgi?cmd=Retrieve&db=pubmed&dopt=Abstract&list_uids=9037578

- **Bruxism secondary to chronic antidopaminergic drug exposure.**
  Author(s): Micheli F, Fernandez Pardal M, Gatto M, Asconape J, Giannaula R, Parera IC.
  Source: Clinical Neuropharmacology. 1993 August; 16(4): 315-23.
  http://www.ncbi.nlm.nih.gov/entrez/query.fcgi?cmd=Retrieve&db=pubmed&dopt=Abstract&list_uids=8104096

- **Bruxism splints: a laboratory viewpoint.**
  Author(s): Weinhardt J.
  Source: Dent Lab Rev. 1985 June; 60(6): 11-2, 14, 16. No Abstract Available.
  http://www.ncbi.nlm.nih.gov/entrez/query.fcgi?cmd=Retrieve&db=pubmed&dopt=Abstract&list_uids=3860425

- **Bruxism the undercover crunch.**
  Author(s): Budds JM.
  Source: Dental Assistant (Chicago, Ill. : 1994). 1976 April; 45(4): 21-3.
  http://www.ncbi.nlm.nih.gov/entrez/query.fcgi?cmd=Retrieve&db=pubmed&dopt=Abstract&list_uids=1074375

- **Bruxism threshold: an explanation for successful treatment of the multifactorial aetiology of bruxism.**
  Author(s): Nel JC, Bester SP, Snyman WD.
  Source: Aust Prosthodont J. 1995; 9: 33-7. Review.
  http://www.ncbi.nlm.nih.gov/entrez/query.fcgi?cmd=Retrieve&db=pubmed&dopt=Abstract&list_uids=9063132

- **Bruxism, neck pain, and a history of child sexual abuse.**
  Author(s): Messer AA.
  Source: J Med Assoc Ga. 1992 November; 81(11): 637-40. No Abstract Available.
  http://www.ncbi.nlm.nih.gov/entrez/query.fcgi?cmd=Retrieve&db=pubmed&dopt=Abstract&list_uids=1431654

- **Bruxism, pulpal pain and restorative material.**
  Author(s): Scimone FS.
  Source: Dent Surv. 1976 September; 52(9): 62-3. No Abstract Available.
  http://www.ncbi.nlm.nih.gov/entrez/query.fcgi?cmd=Retrieve&db=pubmed&dopt=Abstract&list_uids=1074492

- **Bruxism.**
  Author(s): Scally KB, Knox GA, Archer M.
  Source: Aust Dent J. 1991 October; 36(5): 406. No Abstract Available.
  http://www.ncbi.nlm.nih.gov/entrez/query.fcgi?cmd=Retrieve&db=pubmed&dopt=Abstract&list_uids=1755763

- **Bruxism.**
  Author(s): Jacome DE.
  Source: Neurology. 1990 April; 40(4): 727-8.
  http://www.ncbi.nlm.nih.gov/entrez/query.fcgi?cmd=Retrieve&db=pubmed&dopt=Abstract&list_uids=2320262

- **Bruxism.**
  Author(s): Scharer P.
  Source: Front Oral Physiol. 1974; 1(0): 293-322. Review. No Abstract Available.
  http://www.ncbi.nlm.nih.gov/entrez/query.fcgi?cmd=Retrieve&db=pubmed&dopt=Abstract&list_uids=4609874

- **Bruxism: a review and clinical approach to treatment.**
  Author(s): Schulte JK.
  Source: Northwest Dent. 1982 September-October; 61(5): 13-8. Review. No Abstract Available.
  http://www.ncbi.nlm.nih.gov/entrez/query.fcgi?cmd=Retrieve&db=pubmed&dopt=Abstract&list_uids=6755385

- **Bruxism: a review of the literature. Part I.**
  Author(s): Faulkner KD.
  Source: Aust Dent J. 1990 June; 35(3): 266-76. Review.
  http://www.ncbi.nlm.nih.gov/entrez/query.fcgi?cmd=Retrieve&db=pubmed&dopt=Abstract&list_uids=2203332

- **Bruxism: a review of the literature. Part II.**
  Author(s): Faulkner KD.
  Source: Aust Dent J. 1990 August; 35(4): 355-61. Review.
  http://www.ncbi.nlm.nih.gov/entrez/query.fcgi?cmd=Retrieve&db=pubmed&dopt=Abstract&list_uids=2152762

- **Bruxism: a worn out concept.**
  Author(s): Scally KB.
  Source: Cranio. 1991 July; 9(3): 183-5. No Abstract Available.
  http://www.ncbi.nlm.nih.gov/entrez/query.fcgi?cmd=Retrieve&db=pubmed&dopt=Abstract&list_uids=1810661

- **Bruxism: aetiology, clinical signs and symptoms.**
  Author(s): Kleinberg I.
  Source: Aust Prosthodont J. 1994; 8: 9-17. Review.
  http://www.ncbi.nlm.nih.gov/entrez/query.fcgi?cmd=Retrieve&db=pubmed&dopt=Abstract&list_uids=8611311

- **Bruxism: emotional symptom or dental occlusal problem?**
  Author(s): Detsch SG.
  Source: Us Navy Med. 1978 March; 69(3): 26-9. Review. No Abstract Available.
  http://www.ncbi.nlm.nih.gov/entrez/query.fcgi?cmd=Retrieve&db=pubmed&dopt=Abstract&list_uids=366944

- **Bruxism: its significance in coma.**
  Author(s): Pratap-Chand R, Gourie-Devi M.
  Source: Clinical Neurology and Neurosurgery. 1985; 87(2): 113-7.
  http://www.ncbi.nlm.nih.gov/entrez/query.fcgi?cmd=Retrieve&db=pubmed&dopt=Abstract&list_uids=4028585

- **Bruxism: the changing situation.**
  Author(s): Shepherd RW, Price AS.
  Source: Aust Dent J. 1971 August; 16(4): 243-8. No Abstract Available.
  http://www.ncbi.nlm.nih.gov/entrez/query.fcgi?cmd=Retrieve&db=pubmed&dopt=Abstract&list_uids=4940672

- **Buspirone as an antidote to SSRI-induced bruxism in 4 cases.**
  Author(s): Bostwick JM, Jaffee MS.
  Source: The Journal of Clinical Psychiatry. 1999 December; 60(12): 857-60.
  http://www.ncbi.nlm.nih.gov/entrez/query.fcgi?cmd=Retrieve&db=pubmed&dopt=Abstract&list_uids=10665633

- **Buspirone as an antidote to venlafaxine-induced bruxism.**
  Author(s): Jaffee MS, Bostwick JM.
  Source: Psychosomatics. 2000 November-December; 41(6): 535-6.
  http://www.ncbi.nlm.nih.gov/entrez/query.fcgi?cmd=Retrieve&db=pubmed&dopt=Abstract&list_uids=11110119

- **Can bruxism respond to serotonin reuptake inhibitors?**
  Author(s): Stein DJ, Van Greunen G, Niehaus D.
  Source: The Journal of Clinical Psychiatry. 1998 March; 59(3): 133.
  http://www.ncbi.nlm.nih.gov/entrez/query.fcgi?cmd=Retrieve&db=pubmed&dopt=Abstract&list_uids=9541159

- **Causes, manifestations, and management of severe intractable and stereotyped bruxism.**
  Author(s): Myers DE.
  Source: Tmj Update. 1990 January-February; 8(1): 1, 14-6. No Abstract Available.
  http://www.ncbi.nlm.nih.gov/entrez/query.fcgi?cmd=Retrieve&db=pubmed&dopt=Abstract&list_uids=2077633

- **Changes in self-reported incidence of nocturnal bruxism in college students: 1966-2002.**
  Author(s): Granada S, Hicks RA.
  Source: Percept Mot Skills. 2003 December; 97(3 Pt 1): 777-8. Review.
  http://www.ncbi.nlm.nih.gov/entrez/query.fcgi?cmd=Retrieve&db=pubmed&dopt=Abstract&list_uids=14738339

- **Changes in the incidence of nocturnal bruxism in college students: 1966-1989.**
  Author(s): Hicks RA, Conti PA.
  Source: Percept Mot Skills. 1989 October; 69(2): 481-2.
  http://www.ncbi.nlm.nih.gov/entrez/query.fcgi?cmd=Retrieve&db=pubmed&dopt=Abstract&list_uids=2812995

- **Chronic headache and nocturnal bruxism in a 5-year-old child treated with an occlusal splint.**
  Author(s): Jones CM.
  Source: International Journal of Paediatric Dentistry / the British Paedodontic Society [and] the International Association of Dentistry for Children. 1993 June; 3(2): 95-7.
  http://www.ncbi.nlm.nih.gov/entrez/query.fcgi?cmd=Retrieve&db=pubmed&dopt=Abstract&list_uids=8218118

- **Cigarette smoking and bruxism.**
  Author(s): Madrid G, Madrid S, Vranesh JG, Hicks RA.
  Source: Percept Mot Skills. 1998 December; 87(3 Pt 1): 898.
  http://www.ncbi.nlm.nih.gov/entrez/query.fcgi?cmd=Retrieve&db=pubmed&dopt=Abstract&list_uids=9885057

- **Cigarette smoking as a risk factor or an exacerbating factor for restless legs syndrome and sleep bruxism.**
  Author(s): Lavigne GL, Lobbezoo F, Rompre PH, Nielsen TA, Montplaisir J.
  Source: Sleep. 1997 April; 20(4): 290-3.
  http://www.ncbi.nlm.nih.gov/entrez/query.fcgi?cmd=Retrieve&db=pubmed&dopt=Abstract&list_uids=9231955

- **Citalopram-induced bruxism.**
  Author(s): Wise M.
  Source: The British Journal of Psychiatry; the Journal of Mental Science. 2001 February; 178: 182.
  http://www.ncbi.nlm.nih.gov/entrez/query.fcgi?cmd=Retrieve&db=pubmed&dopt=Abstract&list_uids=11157444

- **Combating the adverse effects of bruxism in one visit.**
  Author(s): Benk J.
  Source: Dent Today. 2004 January; 23(1): 68-71. No Abstract Available.
  http://www.ncbi.nlm.nih.gov/entrez/query.fcgi?cmd=Retrieve&db=pubmed&dopt=Abstract&list_uids=14969000

- **Comparison of MMPI scores with self-report of sleep disturbance and bruxism in the facial pain population.**
  Author(s): Harness DM, Peltier B.
  Source: Cranio. 1992 January; 10(1): 70-4.
  http://www.ncbi.nlm.nih.gov/entrez/query.fcgi?cmd=Retrieve&db=pubmed&dopt=Abstract&list_uids=1302654

- **Computer analysis of nocturnal tooth-contact patterns in relation to bruxism and mandibular joint dysfunction in man.**
  Author(s): Trenouth MJ.
  Source: Archives of Oral Biology. 1978; 23(9): 821-4.
  http://www.ncbi.nlm.nih.gov/entrez/query.fcgi?cmd=Retrieve&db=pubmed&dopt=Abstract&list_uids=299022

- **Contingent electrical lip stimulation for sleep bruxism: a pilot study.**
  Author(s): Nishigawa K, Kondo K, Takeuchi H, Clark GT.
  Source: The Journal of Prosthetic Dentistry. 2003 April; 89(4): 412-7.
  http://www.ncbi.nlm.nih.gov/entrez/query.fcgi?cmd=Retrieve&db=pubmed&dopt=Abstract&list_uids=12690356

- **Criteria for the detection of sleep-associated bruxism in humans.**
  Author(s): Ikeda T, Nishigawa K, Kondo K, Takeuchi H, Clark GT.
  Source: J Orofac Pain. 1996 Summer; 10(3): 270-82.
  http://www.ncbi.nlm.nih.gov/entrez/query.fcgi?cmd=Retrieve&db=pubmed&dopt=Abstract&list_uids=9161232

- **Decreased amount of slow wave sleep in nocturnal bruxism is not improved by dental splint therapy.**
  Author(s): Nagels G, Okkerse W, Braem M, Van Bogaert PP, De Deyn B, Poirrier R, De Deyn PP.
  Source: Acta Neurol Belg. 2001 September; 101(3): 152-9.
  http://www.ncbi.nlm.nih.gov/entrez/query.fcgi?cmd=Retrieve&db=pubmed&dopt=Abstract&list_uids=11817263

- **Dental erosion and bruxism. A tooth wear analysis from south east Queensland.**
  Author(s): Khan F, Young WG, Daley TJ.
  Source: Aust Dent J. 1998 April; 43(2): 117-27.
  http://www.ncbi.nlm.nih.gov/entrez/query.fcgi?cmd=Retrieve&db=pubmed&dopt=Abstract&list_uids=9612986

- **Descriptive physiological data on a sleep bruxism population.**
  Author(s): Bader GG, Kampe T, Tagdae T, Karlsson S, Blomqvist M.
  Source: Sleep. 1997 November; 20(11): 982-90.
  http://www.ncbi.nlm.nih.gov/entrez/query.fcgi?cmd=Retrieve&db=pubmed&dopt=Abstract&list_uids=9456463

- **Destructive bruxism: sleep stage relationship.**
  Author(s): Ware JC, Rugh JD.
  Source: Sleep. 1988 April; 11(2): 172-81.
  http://www.ncbi.nlm.nih.gov/entrez/query.fcgi?cmd=Retrieve&db=pubmed&dopt=Abstract&list_uids=3381058

- **Development of a portable bruxism monitoring and analysis device equipped with a microcomputer and its practical application.**
  Author(s): Sakagami R, Horii T, Ino S, Matoba K, Kato H, Kawanami M.
  Source: Frontiers of Medical and Biological Engineering : the International Journal of the Japan Society of Medical Electronics and Biological Engineering. 2002; 11(4): 295-306.
  http://www.ncbi.nlm.nih.gov/entrez/query.fcgi?cmd=Retrieve&db=pubmed&dopt=Abstract&list_uids=12735429

- **Diagnosis and treatment of bruxism: a review of the literature.**
  Author(s): Gallagher SJ.
  Source: Gen Dent. 1980 March-April; 28(2): 62-5. Review. No Abstract Available.
  http://www.ncbi.nlm.nih.gov/entrez/query.fcgi?cmd=Retrieve&db=pubmed&dopt=Abstract&list_uids=7005020

- **Distribution of muscle activity during sleep in bruxism.**
  Author(s): Wieselmann G, Permann R, Korner E, Flooh E, Reinhart B, Moser F, Lechner H.
  Source: European Neurology. 1986; 25 Suppl 2: 111-6.
  http://www.ncbi.nlm.nih.gov/entrez/query.fcgi?cmd=Retrieve&db=pubmed&dopt=Abstract&list_uids=3758113

- **Do bruxism and temporomandibular disorders have a cause-and-effect relationship?**
  Author(s): Lobbezoo F, Lavigne GJ.
  Source: J Orofac Pain. 1997 Winter; 11(1): 15-23. Review.
  http://www.ncbi.nlm.nih.gov/entrez/query.fcgi?cmd=Retrieve&db=pubmed&dopt=Abstract&list_uids=10332307

- **Does tooth wear status predict ongoing sleep bruxism in 30-year-old Japanese subjects?**
  Author(s): Baba K, Haketa T, Clark GT, Ohyama T.
  Source: Int J Prosthodont. 2004 January-February; 17(1): 39-44.
  http://www.ncbi.nlm.nih.gov/entrez/query.fcgi?cmd=Retrieve&db=pubmed&dopt=Abstract&list_uids=15008231

- **Double-blind, crossover, placebo-controlled trial of bromocriptine in patients with sleep bruxism.**
  Author(s): Lavigne GJ, Soucy JP, Lobbezoo F, Manzini C, Blanchet PJ, Montplaisir JY.
  Source: Clinical Neuropharmacology. 2001 May-June; 24(3): 145-9.
  http://www.ncbi.nlm.nih.gov/entrez/query.fcgi?cmd=Retrieve&db=pubmed&dopt=Abstract&list_uids=11391125

- **Drugs and bruxism: a critical review.**
  Author(s): Winocur E, Gavish A, Voikovitch M, Emodi-Perlman A, Eli I.
  Source: J Orofac Pain. 2003 Spring; 17(2): 99-111.
  http://www.ncbi.nlm.nih.gov/entrez/query.fcgi?cmd=Retrieve&db=pubmed&dopt=Abstract&list_uids=12836498

- **EEG checkerboard pattern of bruxism.**
  Author(s): Hirsch LJ, Crispin D.
  Source: Neurology. 1999 September 11; 53(4): 669.
  http://www.ncbi.nlm.nih.gov/entrez/query.fcgi?cmd=Retrieve&db=pubmed&dopt=Abstract&list_uids=10489024

- **Effect of a full-arch maxillary occlusal splint on parafunctional activity during sleep in patients with nocturnal bruxism and signs and symptoms of craniomandibular disorders.**
  Author(s): Holmgren K, Sheikholeslam A, Riise C.
  Source: The Journal of Prosthetic Dentistry. 1993 March; 69(3): 293-7.
  http://www.ncbi.nlm.nih.gov/entrez/query.fcgi?cmd=Retrieve&db=pubmed&dopt=Abstract&list_uids=8445561

- **Effect of occlusal splints on the EMG activity of masseter and temporal muscles in bruxism with clinical symptoms.**
  Author(s): Hamada T, Kotani H, Kawazoe Y, Yamada S.
  Source: Journal of Oral Rehabilitation. 1982 March; 9(2): 119-23.
  http://www.ncbi.nlm.nih.gov/entrez/query.fcgi?cmd=Retrieve&db=pubmed&dopt=Abstract&list_uids=6951020

- **Effectiveness of arousal and arousal plus overcorrection to reduce nocturnal bruxism.**
  Author(s): Watson TS.
  Source: Journal of Behavior Therapy and Experimental Psychiatry. 1993 June; 24(2): 181-5.
  http://www.ncbi.nlm.nih.gov/entrez/query.fcgi?cmd=Retrieve&db=pubmed&dopt=Abstract&list_uids=8263225

- **Effects of bruxism: a review of the literature.**
  Author(s): Glaros AG, Rao SM.
  Source: The Journal of Prosthetic Dentistry. 1977 August; 38(2): 149-57. Review.
  http://www.ncbi.nlm.nih.gov/entrez/query.fcgi?cmd=Retrieve&db=pubmed&dopt=Abstract&list_uids=330842

- **Effects of canine versus molar occlusal splint guidance on nocturnal bruxism and craniomandibular symptomatology.**
  Author(s): Rugh JD, Graham GS, Smith JC, Ohrbach RK.
  Source: J Craniomandib Disord. 1989 Fall; 3(4): 203-10.
  http://www.ncbi.nlm.nih.gov/entrez/query.fcgi?cmd=Retrieve&db=pubmed&dopt=Abstract&list_uids=2639157

- **Effects of the D2 receptor agonist bromocriptine on sleep bruxism: report of two single-patient clinical trials.**
  Author(s): Lobbezoo F, Soucy JP, Hartman NG, Montplaisir JY, Lavigne GJ.
  Source: Journal of Dental Research. 1997 September; 76(9): 1610-4.
  http://www.ncbi.nlm.nih.gov/entrez/query.fcgi?cmd=Retrieve&db=pubmed&dopt=Abstract&list_uids=9294496

- **Efficacy of the nocturnal bite plate in the control of bruxism for 3 to 5 year old children.**
  Author(s): Hachmann A, Martins EA, Araujo FB, Nunes R.
  Source: J Clin Pediatr Dent. 1999 Fall; 24(1): 9-15.
  http://www.ncbi.nlm.nih.gov/entrez/query.fcgi?cmd=Retrieve&db=pubmed&dopt=Abstract&list_uids=10709536

- **Ethnicity and bruxism.**
  Author(s): Hicks RA, Lucero-Gorman K, Bautista J, Hicks GJ.
  Source: Percept Mot Skills. 1999 February; 88(1): 240-1.
  http://www.ncbi.nlm.nih.gov/entrez/query.fcgi?cmd=Retrieve&db=pubmed&dopt=Abstract&list_uids=10214650

- **Evaluation of sleep bruxism by polysomnographic analysis in patients with dental implants.**
  Author(s): Tosun T, Karabuda C, Cuhadaroglu C.
  Source: Int J Oral Maxillofac Implants. 2003 March-April; 18(2): 286-92.
  http://www.ncbi.nlm.nih.gov/entrez/query.fcgi?cmd=Retrieve&db=pubmed&dopt=Abstract&list_uids=12705309

- **Evidence that experimentally induced sleep bruxism is a consequence of transient arousal.**
  Author(s): Kato T, Montplaisir JY, Guitard F, Sessle BJ, Lund JP, Lavigne GJ.
  Source: Journal of Dental Research. 2003 April; 82(4): 284-8.
  http://www.ncbi.nlm.nih.gov/entrez/query.fcgi?cmd=Retrieve&db=pubmed&dopt=Abstract&list_uids=12651932

- **Experimental aggression and bruxism in rats.**
  Author(s): Pohto P.
  Source: Acta Odontologica Scandinavica. 1979; 37(2): 117-26.
  http://www.ncbi.nlm.nih.gov/entrez/query.fcgi?cmd=Retrieve&db=pubmed&dopt=Abstract&list_uids=220835

- **Experimental occlusal discrepancies and nocturnal bruxism.**
  Author(s): Rugh JD, Barghi N, Drago CJ.
  Source: The Journal of Prosthetic Dentistry. 1984 April; 51(4): 548-53.
  http://www.ncbi.nlm.nih.gov/entrez/query.fcgi?cmd=Retrieve&db=pubmed&dopt=Abstract&list_uids=6587078

- **Extinction of bruxism by massed practice therapy. Report of case.**
  Author(s): Ayer WA, Gale EN.
  Source: Journal (Canadian Dental Association). 1969 September; 35(9): 492-4.
  http://www.ncbi.nlm.nih.gov/entrez/query.fcgi?cmd=Retrieve&db=pubmed&dopt=Abstract&list_uids=5259363

- **Facial pain and internal pressure of masseter muscle in experimental bruxism in man.**
  Author(s): Christensen LV.
  Source: Archives of Oral Biology. 1971 September; 16(9): 1021-31.
  http://www.ncbi.nlm.nih.gov/entrez/query.fcgi?cmd=Retrieve&db=pubmed&dopt=Abstract&list_uids=5293403

- **Facts about dental bruxism.**
  Author(s): Nadler SC.
  Source: N Y J Dent. 1973 May; 43(5): 153. No Abstract Available.
  http://www.ncbi.nlm.nih.gov/entrez/query.fcgi?cmd=Retrieve&db=pubmed&dopt=Abstract&list_uids=4512032

- **Familial nocturnal facio-mandibular myoclonus mimicking sleep bruxism.**
  Author(s): Vetrugno R, Provini F, Plazzi G, Lombardi C, Liguori R, Lugaresi E, Montagna P.
  Source: Neurology. 2002 February 26; 58(4): 644-7.
  http://www.ncbi.nlm.nih.gov/entrez/query.fcgi?cmd=Retrieve&db=pubmed&dopt=Abstract&list_uids=11865148

- **Further studies of some masticatory characteristics of bruxism.**
  Author(s): Faulkner KD.
  Source: Journal of Oral Rehabilitation. 1990 July; 17(4): 359-64.
  http://www.ncbi.nlm.nih.gov/entrez/query.fcgi?cmd=Retrieve&db=pubmed&dopt=Abstract&list_uids=2213331

- **Habitual snoring and sleep bruxism in a paediatric outpatient population in Hong Kong.**
  Author(s): Ng DK, Kwok KL, Poon G, Chau KW.
  Source: Singapore Med J. 2002 November; 43(11): 554-6.
  http://www.ncbi.nlm.nih.gov/entrez/query.fcgi?cmd=Retrieve&db=pubmed&dopt=Abstract&list_uids=12683350

- **Hostility in TMD/bruxism patients and controls: a clinical comparison study and preliminary results.**
  Author(s): Molina OF, dos Santos J Jr.
  Source: Cranio. 2002 October; 20(4): 282-8.
  http://www.ncbi.nlm.nih.gov/entrez/query.fcgi?cmd=Retrieve&db=pubmed&dopt=Abstract&list_uids=12403186

- **Idiopathic myoclonus in the oromandibular region during sleep: a possible source of confusion in sleep bruxism diagnosis.**
  Author(s): Kato T, Montplaisir JY, Blanchet PJ, Lund JP, Lavigne GJ.
  Source: Movement Disorders : Official Journal of the Movement Disorder Society. 1999 September; 14(5): 865-71.
  http://www.ncbi.nlm.nih.gov/entrez/query.fcgi?cmd=Retrieve&db=pubmed&dopt=Abstract&list_uids=10495054

- **Impact of nocturnal bruxism on mercury uptake from dental amalgams.**
  Author(s): Isacsson G, Barregard L, Selden A, Bodin L.
  Source: European Journal of Oral Sciences. 1997 June; 105(3): 251-7.
  http://www.ncbi.nlm.nih.gov/entrez/query.fcgi?cmd=Retrieve&db=pubmed&dopt=Abstract&list_uids=9249192

- **Incidence of bruxism.**
  Author(s): Reding GR, Rubright WC, Zimmerman SO.
  Source: Journal of Dental Research. 1966 July-August; 45(4): 1198-204.
  http://www.ncbi.nlm.nih.gov/entrez/query.fcgi?cmd=Retrieve&db=pubmed&dopt=Abstract&list_uids=5224088

- **Incidence of diurnal and nocturnal bruxism.**
  Author(s): Glaros AG.
  Source: The Journal of Prosthetic Dentistry. 1981 May; 45(5): 545-9.
  http://www.ncbi.nlm.nih.gov/entrez/query.fcgi?cmd=Retrieve&db=pubmed&dopt=Abstract&list_uids=6938686

- **Increases in nocturnal bruxism among college students implicate stress.**
  Author(s): Hicks RA, Conti PA, Bragg HR.
  Source: Medical Hypotheses. 1990 December; 33(4): 239-40.
  http://www.ncbi.nlm.nih.gov/entrez/query.fcgi?cmd=Retrieve&db=pubmed&dopt=Abstract&list_uids=2090924

- **Influence of a bite-plane according to Jeanmonod, on bruxism activity during sleep.**
  Author(s): Okkerse W, Brebels A, De Deyn PP, Nagels G, De Deyn B, Van Bogaert PP, Braem M.
  Source: Journal of Oral Rehabilitation. 2002 October; 29(10): 980-5.
  http://www.ncbi.nlm.nih.gov/entrez/query.fcgi?cmd=Retrieve&db=pubmed&dopt=Abstract&list_uids=12421329

- **Influence of nocturnal bruxism on the stomatognathic system. Part I: a new device for measuring mandibular movements during sleep.**
  Author(s): Amemori Y, Yamashita S, Ai M, Shinoda H, Sato M, Takahashi J.
  Source: Journal of Oral Rehabilitation. 2001 October; 28(10): 943-9.
  http://www.ncbi.nlm.nih.gov/entrez/query.fcgi?cmd=Retrieve&db=pubmed&dopt=Abstract&list_uids=11737566

- **Internal resorption: a case presentation with bruxism as the possible etiology.**
  Author(s): Tindol JE.
  Source: Tex Dent J. 1992 October; 109(10): 13-5. No Abstract Available.
  http://www.ncbi.nlm.nih.gov/entrez/query.fcgi?cmd=Retrieve&db=pubmed&dopt=Abstract&list_uids=1292148

- **Interpret your X-rays. Bruxism.**
  Author(s): Surveyor AB.
  Source: J Indian Dent Assoc. 1985 April; 57(4): 125, 141. No Abstract Available.
  http://www.ncbi.nlm.nih.gov/entrez/query.fcgi?cmd=Retrieve&db=pubmed&dopt=Abstract&list_uids=3867705

- **Intraoral occlusal telemetry. 3. Tooth contacts in chewing, swallowing and bruxism.**
  Author(s): Pameijer JH, Glickman I, Roeber FW.
  Source: J Periodontol. 1969 May; 40(5): 253-8. No Abstract Available.
  http://www.ncbi.nlm.nih.gov/entrez/query.fcgi?cmd=Retrieve&db=pubmed&dopt=Abstract&list_uids=5255338

- **Is bruxism severity a predictor of oral splint efficacy in patients with myofascial face pain?**
  Author(s): Raphael KG, Marbach JJ, Klausner JJ, Teaford MF, Fischoff DK.
  Source: Journal of Oral Rehabilitation. 2003 January; 30(1): 17-29.
  http://www.ncbi.nlm.nih.gov/entrez/query.fcgi?cmd=Retrieve&db=pubmed&dopt=Abstract&list_uids=12485379

- **Liver and kidney foreign bodies granulomatosis in a patient with malocclusion, bruxism, and worn dental prostheses.**
  Author(s): Ballestri M, Baraldi A, Gatti AM, Furci L, Bagni A, Loria P, Rapana RM, Carulli N, Albertazzi A.
  Source: Gastroenterology. 2001 November; 121(5): 1234-8. Erratum In: Gastroenterology 2001 December; 121(6): 1531.
  http://www.ncbi.nlm.nih.gov/entrez/query.fcgi?cmd=Retrieve&db=pubmed&dopt=Abstract&list_uids=11677217

- **Lower number of K-complexes and K-alphas in sleep bruxism: a controlled quantitative study.**
  Author(s): Lavigne GJ, Rompre PH, Guitard F, Sessle BJ, Kato T, Montplaisir JY.
  Source: Clinical Neurophysiology : Official Journal of the International Federation of Clinical Neurophysiology. 2002 May; 113(5): 686-93.
  http://www.ncbi.nlm.nih.gov/entrez/query.fcgi?cmd=Retrieve&db=pubmed&dopt=Abstract&list_uids=11976048

- **Maintaining immediate posterior disclusion on an occlusal splint for patient with severe bruxism habit.**
  Author(s): Davis CR.
  Source: The Journal of Prosthetic Dentistry. 1996 March; 75(3): 338-9.
  http://www.ncbi.nlm.nih.gov/entrez/query.fcgi?cmd=Retrieve&db=pubmed&dopt=Abstract&list_uids=8648585

- **Management of bruxism.**
  Author(s): Guevara AN.
  Source: J Philipp Dent Assoc. 1998 June-August; 50(1): 39-43. No Abstract Available.
  http://www.ncbi.nlm.nih.gov/entrez/query.fcgi?cmd=Retrieve&db=pubmed&dopt=Abstract&list_uids=10202516

- **Managing bruxism and temporomandibular disorders using a centric relation occlusal device.**
  Author(s): Nassif NJ, al-Ghamdi KS.
  Source: Compend Contin Educ Dent. 1999 November; 20(11): 1071-4,1076,1078 Passim; Quiz 1086.
  http://www.ncbi.nlm.nih.gov/entrez/query.fcgi?cmd=Retrieve&db=pubmed&dopt=Abstract&list_uids=10650392

- **Mandibular exercises to control bruxism and deviation problems.**
  Author(s): Quinn JH.
  Source: Cranio. 1995 January; 13(1): 30-4.
  http://www.ncbi.nlm.nih.gov/entrez/query.fcgi?cmd=Retrieve&db=pubmed&dopt=Abstract&list_uids=7585999

- **Masseter muscle nodule due to bruxism. A case in point.**
  Author(s): Shuren S.
  Source: Oral Surg Oral Med Oral Pathol. 1986 August; 62(2): 140-1.
  http://www.ncbi.nlm.nih.gov/entrez/query.fcgi?cmd=Retrieve&db=pubmed&dopt=Abstract&list_uids=3489214

- **Mast cells in masseter muscle in experimental bruxism in man.**
  Author(s): Christensen LV.
  Source: Journal of Oral Rehabilitation. 1978 January; 5(1): 23-7.
  http://www.ncbi.nlm.nih.gov/entrez/query.fcgi?cmd=Retrieve&db=pubmed&dopt=Abstract&list_uids=272440

- **Methodological considerations concerning the use of Bruxcore Plates to evaluate nocturnal bruxism.**
  Author(s): Pierce CJ, Gale EN.
  Source: Journal of Dental Research. 1989 June; 68(6): 1110-4.
  http://www.ncbi.nlm.nih.gov/entrez/query.fcgi?cmd=Retrieve&db=pubmed&dopt=Abstract&list_uids=2808870

- **Monitoring bruxism.**
  Author(s): Stock P, Clarke NG.
  Source: Medical & Biological Engineering & Computing. 1983 May; 21(3): 295-300.
  http://www.ncbi.nlm.nih.gov/entrez/query.fcgi?cmd=Retrieve&db=pubmed&dopt=Abstract&list_uids=6876903

- **Motor activity in sleep bruxism with concomitant jaw muscle pain. A retrospective pilot study.**
  Author(s): Lavigne GJ, Rompre PH, Montplaisir JY, Lobbezoo F.
  Source: European Journal of Oral Sciences. 1997 February; 105(1): 92-5.
  http://www.ncbi.nlm.nih.gov/entrez/query.fcgi?cmd=Retrieve&db=pubmed&dopt=Abstract&list_uids=9085035

- **Neurobiological mechanisms involved in sleep bruxism.**
  Author(s): Lavigne GJ, Kato T, Kolta A, Sessle BJ.
  Source: Critical Reviews in Oral Biology and Medicine : an Official Publication of the American Association of Oral Biologists. 2003; 14(1): 30-46. Review.
  http://www.ncbi.nlm.nih.gov/entrez/query.fcgi?cmd=Retrieve&db=pubmed&dopt=Abstract&list_uids=12764018

- **Nocturnal bruxism and its clinical management.**
  Author(s): Attanasio R.
  Source: Dent Clin North Am. 1991 January; 35(1): 245-52. Review.
  http://www.ncbi.nlm.nih.gov/entrez/query.fcgi?cmd=Retrieve&db=pubmed&dopt=Abstract&list_uids=1997355

- **Nocturnal bruxism and self reports of stress-related symptoms.**
  Author(s): Hicks RA, Conti P.
  Source: Percept Mot Skills. 1991 June; 72(3 Pt 2): 1182.
  http://www.ncbi.nlm.nih.gov/entrez/query.fcgi?cmd=Retrieve&db=pubmed&dopt=Abstract&list_uids=1961666

- **Nocturnal bruxism and sleep stages.**
  Author(s): Shafagh K, Hutchins M.
  Source: J Gt Houst Dent Soc. 1992 September; 64(2): 8-10. No Abstract Available.
  http://www.ncbi.nlm.nih.gov/entrez/query.fcgi?cmd=Retrieve&db=pubmed&dopt=Abstract&list_uids=1288574

- **Nocturnal bruxism and type A-B behavior in college students.**
  Author(s): Hicks RA, Chancellor C.
  Source: Psychological Reports. 1987 June; 60(3 Pt 2): 1211-4.
  http://www.ncbi.nlm.nih.gov/entrez/query.fcgi?cmd=Retrieve&db=pubmed&dopt=Abstract&list_uids=3628661

- **Nocturnal bruxism treated by massed negative practice. A case study.**
  Author(s): Vasta R, Wortman HA.
  Source: Behavior Modification. 1988 October; 12(4): 618-26.
  http://www.ncbi.nlm.nih.gov/entrez/query.fcgi?cmd=Retrieve&db=pubmed&dopt=Abstract&list_uids=3223892

- **Nocturnal electromyographic evaluation of bruxism patients undergoing short term splint therapy.**
  Author(s): Solberg WK, Clark GT, Rugh JD.
  Source: Journal of Oral Rehabilitation. 1975 July; 2(3): 215-23.
  http://www.ncbi.nlm.nih.gov/entrez/query.fcgi?cmd=Retrieve&db=pubmed&dopt=Abstract&list_uids=1056979

- Occlusal adjustment and myoelectric activity of the jaw elevator muscles in patients with nocturnal bruxism and craniomandibular disorders.
  Author(s): Holmgren K, Sheikholeslam A.
  Source: Scand J Dent Res. 1994 August; 102(4): 238-43.
  http://www.ncbi.nlm.nih.gov/entrez/query.fcgi?cmd=Retrieve&db=pubmed&dopt=Abstract&list_uids=8091124

- Occlusal interferences in children with bruxism.
  Author(s): Lindqvist B.
  Source: Odontol Revy. 1973; 24(2): 141-8. No Abstract Available.
  http://www.ncbi.nlm.nih.gov/entrez/query.fcgi?cmd=Retrieve&db=pubmed&dopt=Abstract&list_uids=4515071

- Occlusal variables, bruxism and temporomandibular disorders: a clinical and kinesiographic assessment.
  Author(s): Tsolka P, Walter JD, Wilson RF, Preiskel HW.
  Source: Journal of Oral Rehabilitation. 1995 December; 22(12): 849-56.
  http://www.ncbi.nlm.nih.gov/entrez/query.fcgi?cmd=Retrieve&db=pubmed&dopt=Abstract&list_uids=9217296

- Occlusion, bruxism, and the mandibular articulation.
  Author(s): Vaughan HC.
  Source: Ann Dent. 1969 March; 28(1): 2-7. No Abstract Available.
  http://www.ncbi.nlm.nih.gov/entrez/query.fcgi?cmd=Retrieve&db=pubmed&dopt=Abstract&list_uids=5251361

- Occurrence of temporomandibular disorder symptoms in healthy young adults with and without evidence of bruxism.
  Author(s): Allen JD, Rivera-Morales WC, Zwemer JD.
  Source: Cranio. 1990 October; 8(4): 312-8.
  http://www.ncbi.nlm.nih.gov/entrez/query.fcgi?cmd=Retrieve&db=pubmed&dopt=Abstract&list_uids=2098193

- Oral jaw behaviors in TMD and bruxism: a comparison study by severity of bruxism.
  Author(s): Molina OF, dos Santos J, Mazzetto M, Nelson S, Nowlin T, Mainieri ET.
  Source: Cranio. 2001 April; 19(2): 114-22.
  http://www.ncbi.nlm.nih.gov/entrez/query.fcgi?cmd=Retrieve&db=pubmed&dopt=Abstract&list_uids=11842862

- Oral splints: the crutches for temporomandibular disorders and bruxism?
  Author(s): Dao TT, Lavigne GJ.
  Source: Critical Reviews in Oral Biology and Medicine : an Official Publication of the American Association of Oral Biologists. 1998; 9(3): 345-61. Review.
  http://www.ncbi.nlm.nih.gov/entrez/query.fcgi?cmd=Retrieve&db=pubmed&dopt=Abstract&list_uids=9715371

- **Periodontal status and bruxism. A comparative study of patients with periodontal disease and occlusal parafunctions.**
  Author(s): Hanamura H, Houston F, Rylander H, Carlsson GE, Haraldson T, Nyman S.
  Source: J Periodontol. 1987 March; 58(3): 173-6.
  http://www.ncbi.nlm.nih.gov/entrez/query.fcgi?cmd=Retrieve&db=pubmed&dopt=Abstract&list_uids=3470500

- **Perioral and dental perception of mechanical stimulus among subjects with and without awareness of bruxism.**
  Author(s): Mantyvaara J, Sjoholm T, Pertovaara A.
  Source: Acta Odontologica Scandinavica. 2000 June; 58(3): 125-8.
  http://www.ncbi.nlm.nih.gov/entrez/query.fcgi?cmd=Retrieve&db=pubmed&dopt=Abstract&list_uids=10933561

- **Permanent bruxism as a manifestation of the oculo-facial syndrome related to systemic Whipple's disease.**
  Author(s): Tison F, Louvet-Giendaj C, Henry P, Lagueny A, Gaujard E.
  Source: Movement Disorders : Official Journal of the Movement Disorder Society. 1992; 7(1): 82-5.
  http://www.ncbi.nlm.nih.gov/entrez/query.fcgi?cmd=Retrieve&db=pubmed&dopt=Abstract&list_uids=1372960

- **Pityriasis rosea, aphthous stomatitis, and bruxism--a possible psychosomatic aetiology.**
  Author(s): Rudolph M.
  Source: Diastema. 1971; 3(2): 21-2. No Abstract Available.
  http://www.ncbi.nlm.nih.gov/entrez/query.fcgi?cmd=Retrieve&db=pubmed&dopt=Abstract&list_uids=5289526

- **Possible paroxetine-induced bruxism.**
  Author(s): Romanelli F, Adler DA, Bungay KM.
  Source: The Annals of Pharmacotherapy. 1996 November; 30(11): 1246-8.
  http://www.ncbi.nlm.nih.gov/entrez/query.fcgi?cmd=Retrieve&db=pubmed&dopt=Abstract&list_uids=8913405

- **Predictors of bruxism, other oral parafunctions, and tooth wear over a 20-year follow-up period.**
  Author(s): Carlsson GE, Egermark I, Magnusson T.
  Source: J Orofac Pain. 2003 Winter; 17(1): 50-7.
  http://www.ncbi.nlm.nih.gov/entrez/query.fcgi?cmd=Retrieve&db=pubmed&dopt=Abstract&list_uids=12756931

- **Preliminary studies of some masticatory characteristics of bruxism.**
  Author(s): Faulkner KD.
  Source: Journal of Oral Rehabilitation. 1989 May; 16(3): 221-7.
  http://www.ncbi.nlm.nih.gov/entrez/query.fcgi?cmd=Retrieve&db=pubmed&dopt=Abstract&list_uids=2746409

- **Prevalence of bruxism awareness in a Sardinian population.**
  Author(s): Melis M, Abou-Atme YS.
  Source: Cranio. 2003 April; 21(2): 144-51.
  http://www.ncbi.nlm.nih.gov/entrez/query.fcgi?cmd=Retrieve&db=pubmed&dopt=Abstract&list_uids=12723861

- **Prevalence of bruxism in patients with different research diagnostic criteria for temporomandibular disorders (RDC/TMD) diagnoses.**
  Author(s): Manfredini D, Cantini E, Romagnoli M, Bosco M.
  Source: Cranio. 2003 October; 21(4): 279-85.
  http://www.ncbi.nlm.nih.gov/entrez/query.fcgi?cmd=Retrieve&db=pubmed&dopt=Abstract&list_uids=14620701

- **Prevalence of modalities of headaches and bruxism among patients with craniomandibular disorder.**
  Author(s): Molina OF, dos Santos J Jr, Nelson SJ, Grossman E.
  Source: Cranio. 1997 October; 15(4): 314-25.
  http://www.ncbi.nlm.nih.gov/entrez/query.fcgi?cmd=Retrieve&db=pubmed&dopt=Abstract&list_uids=9481994

- **Prevalence of nocturnal and diurnal bruxism in patients with psoriasis.**
  Author(s): Kononen M, Siirila HS.
  Source: The Journal of Prosthetic Dentistry. 1988 August; 60(2): 238-41.
  http://www.ncbi.nlm.nih.gov/entrez/query.fcgi?cmd=Retrieve&db=pubmed&dopt=Abstract&list_uids=3172009

- **Prosthesis and bruxism as the risk in the development of periodontal disease.**
  Author(s): Wigdorowicz-Makowerowa N, Panek H, Marek H.
  Source: Proc Eur Prosthodontic Assoc. 1980; : 43-6. No Abstract Available.
  http://www.ncbi.nlm.nih.gov/entrez/query.fcgi?cmd=Retrieve&db=pubmed&dopt=Abstract&list_uids=6755455

- **Psychogenic bruxism: conceptual and experimental views.**
  Author(s): Keith KD.
  Source: J Nebr Dent Assoc. 1977 Autumn; 54(1): 10-4, 23. Review. No Abstract Available.
  http://www.ncbi.nlm.nih.gov/entrez/query.fcgi?cmd=Retrieve&db=pubmed&dopt=Abstract&list_uids=381593

- **Quantitative study of bite force during sleep associated bruxism.**
  Author(s): Nishigawa K, Bando E, Nakano M.
  Source: Journal of Oral Rehabilitation. 2001 May; 28(5): 485-91.
  http://www.ncbi.nlm.nih.gov/entrez/query.fcgi?cmd=Retrieve&db=pubmed&dopt=Abstract&list_uids=11380790

- **Reasons for bruxism and bruxism in children.**
  Author(s): Batirbaygil Y, Tanboga I, Caglayan F.
  Source: Dent. 1987 May; 2(4): 168-80. English, Turkish. No Abstract Available.
  http://www.ncbi.nlm.nih.gov/entrez/query.fcgi?cmd=Retrieve&db=pubmed&dopt=Abstract&list_uids=3304854

- **Reducing severe diurnal bruxism in two profoundly retarded females.**
  Author(s): Blount RL, Drabman RS, Wilson N, Stewart D.
  Source: J Appl Behav Anal. 1982 Winter; 15(4): 565-71.
  http://www.ncbi.nlm.nih.gov/entrez/query.fcgi?cmd=Retrieve&db=pubmed&dopt=Abstract&list_uids=6891381

- **Rehabilitating a patient with bruxism-associated tooth tissue loss: a literature review and case report.**
  Author(s): Yip KH, Chow TW, Chu FC.
  Source: Gen Dent. 2003 January-February; 51(1): 70-4; Quiz 75-6. Review. Erratum In: Gen Dent. 2003 March-April; 51-2.
  http://www.ncbi.nlm.nih.gov/entrez/query.fcgi?cmd=Retrieve&db=pubmed&dopt=Abstract&list_uids=15061339

- **Relationship between allergy and bruxism in patients with myofascial pain-dysfunction syndrome.**
  Author(s): Olson RE, Laskin DM.
  Source: The Journal of the American Dental Association. 1980 February; 100(2): 209-10.
  http://www.ncbi.nlm.nih.gov/entrez/query.fcgi?cmd=Retrieve&db=pubmed&dopt=Abstract&list_uids=6928151

- **Relationship between malocclusion and bruxism in children and adolescents: a review.**
  Author(s): Vanderas AP, Manetas KJ.
  Source: Pediatr Dent. 1995 January-February; 17(1): 7-12. Review.
  http://www.ncbi.nlm.nih.gov/entrez/query.fcgi?cmd=Retrieve&db=pubmed&dopt=Abstract&list_uids=7899111

- **Reliability of a portable electromyographic unit to measure bruxism.**
  Author(s): Rivera-Morales WC, McCall WD Jr.
  Source: The Journal of Prosthetic Dentistry. 1995 February; 73(2): 184-9.
  http://www.ncbi.nlm.nih.gov/entrez/query.fcgi?cmd=Retrieve&db=pubmed&dopt=Abstract&list_uids=7722935

- **Reliability of clinician judgements of bruxism.**
  Author(s): Marbach JJ, Raphael KG, Janal MN, Hirschkorn-Roth R.
  Source: Journal of Oral Rehabilitation. 2003 February; 30(2): 113-8.
  http://www.ncbi.nlm.nih.gov/entrez/query.fcgi?cmd=Retrieve&db=pubmed&dopt=Abstract&list_uids=12535135

- **Reported bruxism and stress experience in media personnel with or without irregular shift work.**
  Author(s): Ahlberg K, Ahlberg J, Kononen M, Partinen M, Lindholm H, Savolainen A.
  Source: Acta Odontologica Scandinavica. 2003 October; 61(5): 315-8.
  http://www.ncbi.nlm.nih.gov/entrez/query.fcgi?cmd=Retrieve&db=pubmed&dopt=Abstract&list_uids=14763785

- **Reported bruxism and stress experience.**
  Author(s): Ahlberg J, Rantala M, Savolainen A, Suvinen T, Nissinen M, Sarna S, Lindholm H, Kononen M.
  Source: Community Dentistry and Oral Epidemiology. 2002 December; 30(6): 405-8.
  http://www.ncbi.nlm.nih.gov/entrez/query.fcgi?cmd=Retrieve&db=pubmed&dopt=Abstract&list_uids=12453110

- **Reports of SSRI-associated bruxism in the family physician's office.**
  Author(s): Lobbezoo F, van Denderen RJ, Verheij JG, Naeije M.
  Source: J Orofac Pain. 2001 Fall; 15(4): 340-6.
  http://www.ncbi.nlm.nih.gov/entrez/query.fcgi?cmd=Retrieve&db=pubmed&dopt=Abstract&list_uids=12400402

- **Restless legs syndrome and sleep bruxism: prevalence and association among Canadians.**
  Author(s): Lavigne GJ, Montplaisir JY.
  Source: Sleep. 1994 December; 17(8): 739-43.
  http://www.ncbi.nlm.nih.gov/entrez/query.fcgi?cmd=Retrieve&db=pubmed&dopt=Abstract&list_uids=7701186

- **Restoring aesthetics and vertical dimension in a bruxism case.**
  Author(s): Landman P.
  Source: Dent Today. 2000 October; 19(10): 80-4. No Abstract Available.
  http://www.ncbi.nlm.nih.gov/entrez/query.fcgi?cmd=Retrieve&db=pubmed&dopt=Abstract&list_uids=12524810

- **Reversible pulpitis with etiology of bruxism.**
  Author(s): Cooke HG.
  Source: Journal of Endodontics. 1982 June; 8(6): 280-1.
  http://www.ncbi.nlm.nih.gov/entrez/query.fcgi?cmd=Retrieve&db=pubmed&dopt=Abstract&list_uids=6955431

- **Risk factors for sleep bruxism in the general population.**
  Author(s): Ohayon MM, Li KK, Guilleminault C.
  Source: Chest. 2001 January; 119(1): 53-61.
  http://www.ncbi.nlm.nih.gov/entrez/query.fcgi?cmd=Retrieve&db=pubmed&dopt=Abstract&list_uids=11157584

- **Risperidol and withdrawal bruxism in Lewy body dementia.**
  Author(s): Shiwach RS, Woods S.
  Source: International Journal of Geriatric Psychiatry. 1998 January; 13(1): 65-6.
  http://www.ncbi.nlm.nih.gov/entrez/query.fcgi?cmd=Retrieve&db=pubmed&dopt=Abstract&list_uids=9489584

- **Severe amphethamine-induced bruxism: treatment with botulinum toxin.**
  Author(s): See SJ, Tan EK.
  Source: Acta Neurologica Scandinavica. 2003 February; 107(2): 161-3.
  http://www.ncbi.nlm.nih.gov/entrez/query.fcgi?cmd=Retrieve&db=pubmed&dopt=Abstract&list_uids=12580870

- **Severe bruxism following basal ganglia infarcts: insights into pathophysiology.**
  Author(s): Tan EK, Chan LL, Chang HM.
  Source: Journal of the Neurological Sciences. 2004 February 15; 217(2): 229-32.
  http://www.ncbi.nlm.nih.gov/entrez/query.fcgi?cmd=Retrieve&db=pubmed&dopt=Abstract&list_uids=14706229

- **Severe bruxism in a demented patient.**
  Author(s): Stewart JT, Thomas JE, Williams LS.
  Source: Southern Medical Journal. 1993 April; 86(4): 476-7.
  http://www.ncbi.nlm.nih.gov/entrez/query.fcgi?cmd=Retrieve&db=pubmed&dopt=Abstract&list_uids=8465232

- **Sleep bruxism as a manifestation of subclinical rapid eye movement sleep behavior disorder.**
  Author(s): Tachibana N, Yamanaka K, Kaji R, Nagamine T, Watatani K, Kimura J, Shibasaki H.
  Source: Sleep. 1994 September; 17(6): 555-8.
  http://www.ncbi.nlm.nih.gov/entrez/query.fcgi?cmd=Retrieve&db=pubmed&dopt=Abstract&list_uids=7809570

- **Sleep bruxism as a motor disorder.**
  Author(s): De Laat A, Macaluso GM.
  Source: Movement Disorders : Official Journal of the Movement Disorder Society. 2002; 17 Suppl 2: S67-9. Review.
  http://www.ncbi.nlm.nih.gov/entrez/query.fcgi?cmd=Retrieve&db=pubmed&dopt=Abstract&list_uids=11836759

- **Sleep bruxism based on self-report in a nationwide twin cohort.**
  Author(s): Hublin C, Kaprio J, Partinen M, Koskenvuo M.
  Source: Journal of Sleep Research. 1998 March; 7(1): 61-7.
  http://www.ncbi.nlm.nih.gov/entrez/query.fcgi?cmd=Retrieve&db=pubmed&dopt=Abstract&list_uids=9613429

- **Sleep bruxism in patients with sleep-disordered breathing.**
  Author(s): Sjoholm TT, Lowe AA, Miyamoto K, Fleetham JA, Ryan CF.
  Source: Archives of Oral Biology. 2000 October; 45(10): 889-96.
  http://www.ncbi.nlm.nih.gov/entrez/query.fcgi?cmd=Retrieve&db=pubmed&dopt=Abstract&list_uids=10973562

- **Sleep bruxism is a disorder related to periodic arousals during sleep.**
  Author(s): Macaluso GM, Guerra P, Di Giovanni G, Boselli M, Parrino L, Terzano MG.
  Source: Journal of Dental Research. 1998 April; 77(4): 565-73.
  http://www.ncbi.nlm.nih.gov/entrez/query.fcgi?cmd=Retrieve&db=pubmed&dopt=Abstract&list_uids=9539459

- **Sleep bruxism: an oromotor activity secondary to micro-arousal.**
  Author(s): Kato T, Rompre P, Montplaisir JY, Sessle BJ, Lavigne GJ.
  Source: Journal of Dental Research. 2001 October; 80(10): 1940-4.
  http://www.ncbi.nlm.nih.gov/entrez/query.fcgi?cmd=Retrieve&db=pubmed&dopt=Abstract&list_uids=11706956

- **Sleep bruxism: issues to chew on.**
  Author(s): Sessle BJ.
  Source: J Orofac Pain. 2003 Summer; 17(3): 187. No Abstract Available.
  http://www.ncbi.nlm.nih.gov/entrez/query.fcgi?cmd=Retrieve&db=pubmed&dopt=A
  bstract&list_uids=14520765

- **Sleep bruxism: validity of clinical research diagnostic criteria in a controlled polysomnographic study.**
  Author(s): Lavigne GJ, Rompre PH, Montplaisir JY.
  Source: Journal of Dental Research. 1996 January; 75(1): 546-52.
  http://www.ncbi.nlm.nih.gov/entrez/query.fcgi?cmd=Retrieve&db=pubmed&dopt=A
  bstract&list_uids=8655758

- **Sleep bruxism--new findings.**
  Author(s): Muzyka BC.
  Source: Pract Proced Aesthet Dent. 2001 April; 13(3): 190. No Abstract Available.
  http://www.ncbi.nlm.nih.gov/entrez/query.fcgi?cmd=Retrieve&db=pubmed&dopt=A
  bstract&list_uids=11360765

- **Sleep-related bruxism and sleep variables: a critical review.**
  Author(s): Wruble MK, Lumley MA, McGlynn FD.
  Source: J Craniomandib Disord. 1989 Summer; 3(3): 152-8. Review.
  http://www.ncbi.nlm.nih.gov/entrez/query.fcgi?cmd=Retrieve&db=pubmed&dopt=A
  bstract&list_uids=2700989

- **Soft thermoplastics in bruxism appliances.**
  Author(s): Anthony TH.
  Source: Trends Tech Contemp Dent Lab. 1995 September; 12(7): 32-6. No Abstract Available.
  http://www.ncbi.nlm.nih.gov/entrez/query.fcgi?cmd=Retrieve&db=pubmed&dopt=A
  bstract&list_uids=9584705

- **SSRI-associated nocturnal bruxism in four patients.**
  Author(s): Ellison JM, Stanziani P.
  Source: The Journal of Clinical Psychiatry. 1993 November; 54(11): 432-4.
  http://www.ncbi.nlm.nih.gov/entrez/query.fcgi?cmd=Retrieve&db=pubmed&dopt=A
  bstract&list_uids=8270587

- **Stress, anticipatory stress, and psychologic measures related to sleep bruxism.**
  Author(s): Pierce CJ, Chrisman K, Bennett ME, Close JM.
  Source: J Orofac Pain. 1995 Winter; 9(1): 51-6.
  http://www.ncbi.nlm.nih.gov/entrez/query.fcgi?cmd=Retrieve&db=pubmed&dopt=A
  bstract&list_uids=7581205

- **Striatal D2 receptor binding in sleep bruxism: a controlled study with iodine-123-iodobenzamide and single-photon-emission computed tomography.**
  Author(s): Lobbezoo F, Soucy JP, Montplaisir JY, Lavigne GJ.
  Source: Journal of Dental Research. 1996 October; 75(10): 1804-10.
  http://www.ncbi.nlm.nih.gov/entrez/query.fcgi?cmd=Retrieve&db=pubmed&dopt=Abstract&list_uids=8955676

- **Study of the relationship of frustration and anxiety to bruxism.**
  Author(s): Thaller JL, Rosen G, Saltzman S.
  Source: J Periodontol. 1967 May-June; 38(3): 193-7. No Abstract Available.
  http://www.ncbi.nlm.nih.gov/entrez/query.fcgi?cmd=Retrieve&db=pubmed&dopt=Abstract&list_uids=5229284

- **Successful electroconvulsive therapy in major depression with fluvoxamine-induced bruxism.**
  Author(s): Miyaoka T, Yasukawa R, Mihara T, Shimizu Y, Tsubouchi K, Maeda T, Mizuno S, Uegaki J, Inagaki T, Horiguchi J, Tachibana H.
  Source: The Journal of Ect. 2003 September; 19(3): 170-2.
  http://www.ncbi.nlm.nih.gov/entrez/query.fcgi?cmd=Retrieve&db=pubmed&dopt=Abstract&list_uids=12972988

- **Survey of bruxism in an institutionalized mentally retarded population.**
  Author(s): Richmond G, Rugh JD, Dolfi R, Wasilewsky JW.
  Source: Am J Ment Defic. 1984 January; 88(4): 418-21.
  http://www.ncbi.nlm.nih.gov/entrez/query.fcgi?cmd=Retrieve&db=pubmed&dopt=Abstract&list_uids=6695964

- **Survey of current therapy: bruxism splints.**
  Author(s): Lester M, Baer PN.
  Source: Periodontal Case Rep. 1989; 11(1): 23-4. No Abstract Available.
  http://www.ncbi.nlm.nih.gov/entrez/query.fcgi?cmd=Retrieve&db=pubmed&dopt=Abstract&list_uids=2629009

- **Teeth grinding, tongue and lip biting in a 24-month-old boy with meningococcal septicaemia. Report of a case.**
  Author(s): Coyne BM, Montague T.
  Source: International Journal of Paediatric Dentistry / the British Paedodontic Society [and] the International Association of Dentistry for Children. 2002 July; 12(4): 277-80.
  http://www.ncbi.nlm.nih.gov/entrez/query.fcgi?cmd=Retrieve&db=pubmed&dopt=Abstract&list_uids=12121539

- **Tension headache and bruxism in the sleep disordered patient.**
  Author(s): Bailey DR.
  Source: Cranio. 1990 April; 8(2): 174-82.
  http://www.ncbi.nlm.nih.gov/entrez/query.fcgi?cmd=Retrieve&db=pubmed&dopt=Abstract&list_uids=2073698

- **The association between wear facets, bruxism, and severity of facial pain in patients with temporomandibular disorders.**
  Author(s): Pergamalian A, Rudy TE, Zaki HS, Greco CM.
  Source: The Journal of Prosthetic Dentistry. 2003 August; 90(2): 194-200.
  http://www.ncbi.nlm.nih.gov/entrez/query.fcgi?cmd=Retrieve&db=pubmed&dopt=Abstract&list_uids=12886214

- **The bruxism appliance and its varied application: outline of procedure.**
  Author(s): Greenwald AS.
  Source: N Y J Dent. 1968 December; 38(10): 443. No Abstract Available.
  http://www.ncbi.nlm.nih.gov/entrez/query.fcgi?cmd=Retrieve&db=pubmed&dopt=Abstract&list_uids=5246303

- **The effect of bruxism on treatment planning for dental implants.**
  Author(s): Misch CE.
  Source: Dent Today. 2002 September; 21(9): 76-81.
  http://www.ncbi.nlm.nih.gov/entrez/query.fcgi?cmd=Retrieve&db=pubmed&dopt=Abstract&list_uids=12271847

- **The effect of catecholamine precursor L-dopa on sleep bruxism: a controlled clinical trial.**
  Author(s): Lobbezoo F, Lavigne GJ, Tanguay R, Montplaisir JY.
  Source: Movement Disorders : Official Journal of the Movement Disorder Society. 1997 January; 12(1): 73-8.
  http://www.ncbi.nlm.nih.gov/entrez/query.fcgi?cmd=Retrieve&db=pubmed&dopt=Abstract&list_uids=8990057

- **The effect of four-week administration of amitriptyline on sleep bruxism. A double-blind crossover clinical study.**
  Author(s): Raigrodski AJ, Christensen LV, Mohamed SE, Gardiner DM.
  Source: Cranio. 2001 January; 19(1): 21-5.
  http://www.ncbi.nlm.nih.gov/entrez/query.fcgi?cmd=Retrieve&db=pubmed&dopt=Abstract&list_uids=11842836

- **The effect of propranolol on sleep bruxism: hypothetical considerations based on a case study.**
  Author(s): Sjoholm TT, Lehtinen I, Piha SJ.
  Source: Clinical Autonomic Research : Official Journal of the Clinical Autonomic Research Society. 1996 February; 6(1): 37-40.
  http://www.ncbi.nlm.nih.gov/entrez/query.fcgi?cmd=Retrieve&db=pubmed&dopt=Abstract&list_uids=8924755

- **The effects of an occlusal splint on the electromyographic activities of the temporal and masseter muscles during maximal clenching in patients with a habit of nocturnal bruxism and signs and symptoms of craniomandibular disorders.**
  Author(s): Holmgren K, Sheikholeslam A, Riise C, Kopp S.
  Source: Journal of Oral Rehabilitation. 1990 September; 17(5): 447-59.
  http://www.ncbi.nlm.nih.gov/entrez/query.fcgi?cmd=Retrieve&db=pubmed&dopt=Abstract&list_uids=2231163

- **The effects of bruxism.**
  Author(s): Nadler SC.
  Source: J Periodontol. 1966 July-August; 37(4): 311-9. No Abstract Available.
  http://www.ncbi.nlm.nih.gov/entrez/query.fcgi?cmd=Retrieve&db=pubmed&dopt=A
  bstract&list_uids=5220897

- **The effects of hard and soft occlusal splints on nocturnal bruxism.**
  Author(s): Okeson JP.
  Source: The Journal of the American Dental Association. 1987 June; 114(6): 788-91.
  http://www.ncbi.nlm.nih.gov/entrez/query.fcgi?cmd=Retrieve&db=pubmed&dopt=A
  bstract&list_uids=3475357

- **The effects of severe bruxism on sleep architecture: a preliminary report.**
  Author(s): Boutros NN, Montgomery MT, Nishioka G, Hatch JP.
  Source: Clin Electroencephalogr. 1993 April; 24(2): 59-62.
  http://www.ncbi.nlm.nih.gov/entrez/query.fcgi?cmd=Retrieve&db=pubmed&dopt=A
  bstract&list_uids=8500248

- **The effects of unilateral and bilateral chewing, empty clenching and simulated bruxism, on the masticatory-parotid salivary reflex in man.**
  Author(s): Anderson DJ, Hector MP, Linden RW.
  Source: Experimental Physiology. 1996 March; 81(2): 305-12.
  http://www.ncbi.nlm.nih.gov/entrez/query.fcgi?cmd=Retrieve&db=pubmed&dopt=A
  bstract&list_uids=8845144

- **The etiology of bruxism.**
  Author(s): Titus T.
  Source: J Nebr Dent Assoc. 1977 Spring; 53(3): 14-6, 37. Review. No Abstract Available.
  http://www.ncbi.nlm.nih.gov/entrez/query.fcgi?cmd=Retrieve&db=pubmed&dopt=A
  bstract&list_uids=381592

- **The importance of bruxism.**
  Author(s): Nadler SC.
  Source: J Oral Med. 1968 October; 23(4): 142-8. No Abstract Available.
  http://www.ncbi.nlm.nih.gov/entrez/query.fcgi?cmd=Retrieve&db=pubmed&dopt=A
  bstract&list_uids=5250493

- **The masseteric silent period following experimental bruxism in subjects wearing acrylic anterior bite planes.**
  Author(s): Cox PJ, Rothwell PS, Duxbury AJ.
  Source: Journal of Oral Rehabilitation. 1983 January; 10(1): 51-5.
  http://www.ncbi.nlm.nih.gov/entrez/query.fcgi?cmd=Retrieve&db=pubmed&dopt=A
  bstract&list_uids=6572239

- **The neurological relationship of bruxism and sleep.**
  Author(s): Tong D.
  Source: Georgetown Dent J. 1973 Winter; 38(2): 24-5. No Abstract Available.
  http://www.ncbi.nlm.nih.gov/entrez/query.fcgi?cmd=Retrieve&db=pubmed&dopt=A
  bstract&list_uids=4519698

- **The relation of bruxism and dermatoglyphics.**
  Author(s): Polat MH, Azak A, Evlioglu G, Malkondu OK, Atasu M.
  Source: J Clin Pediatr Dent. 2000 Spring; 24(3): 191-4.
  http://www.ncbi.nlm.nih.gov/entrez/query.fcgi?cmd=Retrieve&db=pubmed&dopt=Abstract&list_uids=11314141

- **The relationship between bruxism and temporomandibular joint dysfunction as shown by computer analysis of nocturnal tooth contact patterns.**
  Author(s): Trenouth MJ.
  Source: Journal of Oral Rehabilitation. 1979 January; 6(1): 81-7.
  http://www.ncbi.nlm.nih.gov/entrez/query.fcgi?cmd=Retrieve&db=pubmed&dopt=Abstract&list_uids=282418

- **The relationship between occlusal factors and bruxism in permanent and mixed dentition in Turkish children.**
  Author(s): Sari S, Sonmez H.
  Source: J Clin Pediatr Dent. 2001 Spring; 25(3): 191-4.
  http://www.ncbi.nlm.nih.gov/entrez/query.fcgi?cmd=Retrieve&db=pubmed&dopt=Abstract&list_uids=12049076

- **The relationship of bruxism with craniofacial pain and symptoms from the masticatory system in the adult population.**
  Author(s): Ciancaglini R, Gherlone EF, Radaelli G.
  Source: Journal of Oral Rehabilitation. 2001 September; 28(9): 842-8.
  http://www.ncbi.nlm.nih.gov/entrez/query.fcgi?cmd=Retrieve&db=pubmed&dopt=Abstract&list_uids=11580822

- **The social and psychologic factors of bruxism.**
  Author(s): Pingitore G, Chrobak V, Petrie J.
  Source: The Journal of Prosthetic Dentistry. 1991 March; 65(3): 443-6.
  http://www.ncbi.nlm.nih.gov/entrez/query.fcgi?cmd=Retrieve&db=pubmed&dopt=Abstract&list_uids=2056467

- **Therapeutic effects of the plane occlusal splint on signs and symptoms of craniomandibular disorders in patients with nocturnal bruxism.**
  Author(s): Sheikholeslam A, Holmgren K, Riise C.
  Source: Journal of Oral Rehabilitation. 1993 September; 20(5): 473-82.
  http://www.ncbi.nlm.nih.gov/entrez/query.fcgi?cmd=Retrieve&db=pubmed&dopt=Abstract&list_uids=10412468

- **Tooth wear and bruxism: a sleep laboratory investigation.**
  Author(s): Dettmar DM, Shaw RM, Tilley AJ.
  Source: Aust Dent J. 1987 December; 32(6): 421-6. No Abstract Available.
  http://www.ncbi.nlm.nih.gov/entrez/query.fcgi?cmd=Retrieve&db=pubmed&dopt=Abstract&list_uids=3481976

- **Topical review: sleep bruxism and the role of peripheral sensory influences.**
  Author(s): Kato T, Thie NM, Huynh N, Miyawaki S, Lavigne GJ.
  Source: J Orofac Pain. 2003 Summer; 17(3): 191-213. Review.
  http://www.ncbi.nlm.nih.gov/entrez/query.fcgi?cmd=Retrieve&db=pubmed&dopt=Abstract&list_uids=14520766

- **Traumatic bruxism in a mentally retarded child.**
  Author(s): Brown RH.
  Source: N Z Dent J. 1970 January; 66(303): 67-70. No Abstract Available.
  http://www.ncbi.nlm.nih.gov/entrez/query.fcgi?cmd=Retrieve&db=pubmed&dopt=Abstract&list_uids=5270594

- **Treating bruxism and clenching.**
  Author(s): Quinn JH.
  Source: The Journal of the American Dental Association. 2000 June; 131(6): 723.
  http://www.ncbi.nlm.nih.gov/entrez/query.fcgi?cmd=Retrieve&db=pubmed&dopt=Abstract&list_uids=10860318

- **Treating bruxism and clenching.**
  Author(s): Harnick DJ.
  Source: The Journal of the American Dental Association. 2000 April; 131(4): 436.
  http://www.ncbi.nlm.nih.gov/entrez/query.fcgi?cmd=Retrieve&db=pubmed&dopt=Abstract&list_uids=10770004

- **Treating bruxism and clenching.**
  Author(s): Christensen GJ.
  Source: The Journal of the American Dental Association. 2000 February; 131(2): 233-5.
  http://www.ncbi.nlm.nih.gov/entrez/query.fcgi?cmd=Retrieve&db=pubmed&dopt=Abstract&list_uids=10680392

- **Treating bruxism with the habit-reversal technique.**
  Author(s): Rosenbaum MS, Ayllon T.
  Source: Behaviour Research and Therapy. 1981; 19(1): 87-96.
  http://www.ncbi.nlm.nih.gov/entrez/query.fcgi?cmd=Retrieve&db=pubmed&dopt=Abstract&list_uids=7225040

- **Treating severe bruxism with botulinum toxin.**
  Author(s): Tan EK, Jankovic J.
  Source: The Journal of the American Dental Association. 2000 February; 131(2): 211-6.
  http://www.ncbi.nlm.nih.gov/entrez/query.fcgi?cmd=Retrieve&db=pubmed&dopt=Abstract&list_uids=10680389

- **Treatment of bruxism and bruxomania (clinically tested).**
  Author(s): Grozev L, Michailov T.
  Source: Folia Med (Plovdiv). 1999; 41(1): 147-8. No Abstract Available.
  http://www.ncbi.nlm.nih.gov/entrez/query.fcgi?cmd=Retrieve&db=pubmed&dopt=Abstract&list_uids=10462946

- **Treatment of bruxism with botulinum toxin injections.**
  Author(s): Van Zandijcke M, Marchau MM.
  Source: Journal of Neurology, Neurosurgery, and Psychiatry. 1990 June; 53(6): 530.
  http://www.ncbi.nlm.nih.gov/entrez/query.fcgi?cmd=Retrieve&db=pubmed&dopt=Abstract&list_uids=2380736

- **Treatment of root and alveolar bone resorption associated with bruxism.**
  Author(s): Rawlinson A.
  Source: British Dental Journal. 1991 June 22; 170(12): 445-7.
  http://www.ncbi.nlm.nih.gov/entrez/query.fcgi?cmd=Retrieve&db=pubmed&dopt=Abstract&list_uids=2069830

- **Treatment of severe post-traumatic bruxism with botulinum toxin-A: case report.**
  Author(s): Pidcock FS, Wise JM, Christensen JR.
  Source: Journal of Oral and Maxillofacial Surgery : Official Journal of the American Association of Oral and Maxillofacial Surgeons. 2002 January; 60(1): 115-7.
  http://www.ncbi.nlm.nih.gov/entrez/query.fcgi?cmd=Retrieve&db=pubmed&dopt=Abstract&list_uids=11757023

- **Update and literature review of bruxism.**
  Author(s): Van Dongen CA.
  Source: R I Dent J. 1992 Winter; 25(4): 11, 13-4, 6. Review. No Abstract Available.
  http://www.ncbi.nlm.nih.gov/entrez/query.fcgi?cmd=Retrieve&db=pubmed&dopt=Abstract&list_uids=1306910

- **Urinary catecholamine levels and bruxism in children.**
  Author(s): Vanderas AP, Menenakou M, Kouimtzis T, Papagiannoulis L.
  Source: Journal of Oral Rehabilitation. 1999 February; 26(2): 103-10.
  http://www.ncbi.nlm.nih.gov/entrez/query.fcgi?cmd=Retrieve&db=pubmed&dopt=Abstract&list_uids=10080306

- **Utility and validity of a new EMG-based bruxism detection system.**
  Author(s): Haketa T, Baba K, Akishige S, Fueki K, Kino K, Ohyama T.
  Source: Int J Prosthodont. 2003 July-August; 16(4): 422-8.
  http://www.ncbi.nlm.nih.gov/entrez/query.fcgi?cmd=Retrieve&db=pubmed&dopt=Abstract&list_uids=12956499

- **Variability in sleep bruxism activity over time.**
  Author(s): Lavigne GJ, Guitard F, Rompre PH, Montplaisir JY.
  Source: Journal of Sleep Research. 2001 September; 10(3): 237-44.
  http://www.ncbi.nlm.nih.gov/entrez/query.fcgi?cmd=Retrieve&db=pubmed&dopt=Abstract&list_uids=11696077

- **Various methods of achieving restoration of tooth structure loss due to bruxism.**
  Author(s): Nel JC, Marais JT, van Vuuren PA.
  Source: J Esthet Dent. 1996; 8(4): 183-8. No Abstract Available.
  http://www.ncbi.nlm.nih.gov/entrez/query.fcgi?cmd=Retrieve&db=pubmed&dopt=Abstract&list_uids=9468839

CHAPTER 2. ALTERNATIVE MEDICINE AND BRUXISM

Overview

In this chapter, we will begin by introducing you to official information sources on complementary and alternative medicine (CAM) relating to bruxism. At the conclusion of this chapter, we will provide additional sources.

National Center for Complementary and Alternative Medicine

The National Center for Complementary and Alternative Medicine (NCCAM) of the National Institutes of Health (**http://nccam.nih.gov/**) has created a link to the National Library of Medicine's databases to facilitate research for articles that specifically relate to bruxism and complementary medicine. To search the database, go to the following Web site: **http://www.nlm.nih.gov/nccam/camonpubmed.html**. Select "CAM on PubMed." Enter "bruxism" (or synonyms) into the search box. Click "Go." The following references provide information on particular aspects of complementary and alternative medicine that are related to bruxism:

- **A comparison of biofeedback and occlusal adjustment on bruxism.**
  Author(s): Kardachi BJ, Bailey JO, Ash MM.
  Source: J Periodontol. 1978 July; 49(7): 367-72.
  http://www.ncbi.nlm.nih.gov/entrez/query.fcgi?cmd=Retrieve&db=pubmed&dopt=Abstract&list_uids=279664

- **A comparison of different treatments for nocturnal bruxism.**
  Author(s): Pierce CJ, Gale EN.
  Source: Journal of Dental Research. 1988 March; 67(3): 597-601.
  http://www.ncbi.nlm.nih.gov/entrez/query.fcgi?cmd=Retrieve&db=pubmed&dopt=Abstract&list_uids=3170898

- **A comparison of stress-reduction behavioral counseling and contingent nocturnal EMG feedback for the treatment of bruxism.**
  Author(s): Casas JM, Beemsterboer P, Clark GT.

Source: Behaviour Research and Therapy. 1982; 20(1): 9-15.
http://www.ncbi.nlm.nih.gov/entrez/query.fcgi?cmd=Retrieve&db=pubmed&dopt=A
bstract&list_uids=7066007

- **A comparison of the muscular relaxation effect of TENS and EMG-biofeedback in patients with bruxism.**
  Author(s): Wieselmann-Penkner K, Janda M, Lorenzoni M, Polansky R.
  Source: Journal of Oral Rehabilitation. 2001 September; 28(9): 849-53.
  http://www.ncbi.nlm.nih.gov/entrez/query.fcgi?cmd=Retrieve&db=pubmed&dopt=A
  bstract&list_uids=11580823

- **A method to control bruxism: biofeedback-assisted relaxation therapy.**
  Author(s): Cannistraci AJ.
  Source: J Am Soc Prev Dent. 1976 December; 6(6): 12-5. No Abstract Available.
  http://www.ncbi.nlm.nih.gov/entrez/query.fcgi?cmd=Retrieve&db=pubmed&dopt=A
  bstract&list_uids=801902

- **A more efficient biofeedback procedure for the treatment of nocturnal bruxism.**
  Author(s): Moss RA, Hammer D, Adams HE, Jenkins JO, Thompson K, Haber J.
  Source: Journal of Oral Rehabilitation. 1982 March; 9(2): 125-31.
  http://www.ncbi.nlm.nih.gov/entrez/query.fcgi?cmd=Retrieve&db=pubmed&dopt=A
  bstract&list_uids=7040615

- **A review of the literature on, and a discussion of studies of bruxism and its psychogenesis and some new psychological hypotheses.**
  Author(s): Olkinuora M.
  Source: Suom Hammaslaak Toim. 1969; 65(6): 312-24. No Abstract Available.
  http://www.ncbi.nlm.nih.gov/entrez/query.fcgi?cmd=Retrieve&db=pubmed&dopt=A
  bstract&list_uids=5266554

- **An evaluation of bruxism control: massed negative practice and automated relaxation training.**
  Author(s): Heller RF, Forgione AG.
  Source: Journal of Dental Research. 1975 November-December; 54(6): 1120-3.
  http://www.ncbi.nlm.nih.gov/entrez/query.fcgi?cmd=Retrieve&db=pubmed&dopt=A
  bstract&list_uids=1104673

- **Awareness/relaxation training and transcutaneous electrical neural stimulation in the treatment of bruxism.**
  Author(s): Treacy K.
  Source: Journal of Oral Rehabilitation. 1999 April; 26(4): 280-7.
  http://www.ncbi.nlm.nih.gov/entrez/query.fcgi?cmd=Retrieve&db=pubmed&dopt=A
  bstract&list_uids=10232855

- **Battling bruxism through biofeedback.**
  Author(s): Hamilton RA.
  Source: Tic. 1986 May; 45(5): 8-11. No Abstract Available.
  http://www.ncbi.nlm.nih.gov/entrez/query.fcgi?cmd=Retrieve&db=pubmed&dopt=A
  bstract&list_uids=3461580

- **Bruxism as an emotional reactive disturbance.**
  Author(s): Shapiro S, Shanon J.
  Source: Psychosomatics. 1965 November-December; 6(6): 427-30.
  http://www.ncbi.nlm.nih.gov/entrez/query.fcgi?cmd=Retrieve&db=pubmed&dopt=A bstract&list_uids=5845953

- **Bruxism in prison.**
  Author(s): Ciolon PG Jr.
  Source: Rev Odontol P R. 1989 August-October; 27(3): 32-6. No Abstract Available.
  http://www.ncbi.nlm.nih.gov/entrez/query.fcgi?cmd=Retrieve&db=pubmed&dopt=A bstract&list_uids=2700829

- **Bruxism.**
  Author(s): Graf H.
  Source: Dent Clin North Am. 1969 July; 13(3): 659-65. No Abstract Available.
  http://www.ncbi.nlm.nih.gov/entrez/query.fcgi?cmd=Retrieve&db=pubmed&dopt=A bstract&list_uids=5256151

- **Bruxism. How to stop tooth grinding and clenching.**
  Author(s): Leung AK, Robson WL.
  Source: Postgraduate Medicine. 1991 June; 89(8): 167-8, 171.
  http://www.ncbi.nlm.nih.gov/entrez/query.fcgi?cmd=Retrieve&db=pubmed&dopt=A bstract&list_uids=2038589

- **Bruxism: a critical review.**
  Author(s): Glaros AG, Rao SM.
  Source: Psychological Bulletin. 1977 July; 84(4): 767-81. Review.
  http://www.ncbi.nlm.nih.gov/entrez/query.fcgi?cmd=Retrieve&db=pubmed&dopt=A bstract&list_uids=331380

- **Can taste aversion prevent bruxism?**
  Author(s): Nissani M.
  Source: Applied Psychophysiology and Biofeedback. 2000 March; 25(1): 43-54.
  http://www.ncbi.nlm.nih.gov/entrez/query.fcgi?cmd=Retrieve&db=pubmed&dopt=A bstract&list_uids=10832509

- **Controlling bruxism through automated aversive conditioning.**
  Author(s): Heller RF, Strang HR.
  Source: Behaviour Research and Therapy. 1973 August; 11(3): 327-9.
  http://www.ncbi.nlm.nih.gov/entrez/query.fcgi?cmd=Retrieve&db=pubmed&dopt=A bstract&list_uids=4727295

- **Current knowledge on awake and sleep bruxism: overview.**
  Author(s): Kato T, Dal-Fabbro C, Lavigne GJ.
  Source: Alpha Omegan. 2003 July; 96(2): 24-32. Review. No Abstract Available.
  http://www.ncbi.nlm.nih.gov/entrez/query.fcgi?cmd=Retrieve&db=pubmed&dopt=A bstract&list_uids=12955779

- **Effect of occlusal splint and transcutaneous electric nerve stimulation on the signs and symptoms of temporomandibular disorders in patients with bruxism.**
  Author(s): Alvarez-Arenal A, Junquera LM, Fernandez JP, Gonzalez I, Olay S.
  Source: Journal of Oral Rehabilitation. 2002 September; 29(9): 858-63.
  http://www.ncbi.nlm.nih.gov/entrez/query.fcgi?cmd=Retrieve&db=pubmed&dopt=Abstract&list_uids=12366541

- **Effects of psychological techniques on bruxism in children with primary teeth.**
  Author(s): Restrepo CC, Alvarez E, Jaramillo C, Velez C, Valencia I.
  Source: Journal of Oral Rehabilitation. 2001 April; 28(4): 354-60.
  http://www.ncbi.nlm.nih.gov/entrez/query.fcgi?cmd=Retrieve&db=pubmed&dopt=Abstract&list_uids=11350589

- **EMG-activated feedback alarms for the treatment of nocturnal bruxism: current status and future directions.**
  Author(s): Cassisi JE, McGlynn FD, Belles DR.
  Source: Biofeedback Self Regul. 1987 March; 12(1): 13-30. Review.
  http://www.ncbi.nlm.nih.gov/entrez/query.fcgi?cmd=Retrieve&db=pubmed&dopt=Abstract&list_uids=3311171

- **Erosion arising from a nutritional factor with concomitant bruxism. A clinical case report.**
  Author(s): Spanauf AJ.
  Source: Aust Dent J. 1973 August; 18(4): 233-4. No Abstract Available.
  http://www.ncbi.nlm.nih.gov/entrez/query.fcgi?cmd=Retrieve&db=pubmed&dopt=Abstract&list_uids=4520871

- **Factors associated with nocturnal bruxism and its treatment.**
  Author(s): Funch DP, Gale EN.
  Source: Journal of Behavioral Medicine. 1980 December; 3(4): 385-97.
  http://www.ncbi.nlm.nih.gov/entrez/query.fcgi?cmd=Retrieve&db=pubmed&dopt=Abstract&list_uids=7230260

- **Holistic care concepts, bruxism and necrotizing ulcerative gingivitis.**
  Author(s): Pear JH.
  Source: Dent Hyg (Chic). 1982 September; 56(9): 24-9. No Abstract Available.
  http://www.ncbi.nlm.nih.gov/entrez/query.fcgi?cmd=Retrieve&db=pubmed&dopt=Abstract&list_uids=6958589

- **Hypnotherapy in the treatment of the chronic nocturnal use of a dental splint prescribed for bruxism.**
  Author(s): Somer E.
  Source: Int J Clin Exp Hypn. 1991 July; 39(3): 145-54.
  http://www.ncbi.nlm.nih.gov/entrez/query.fcgi?cmd=Retrieve&db=pubmed&dopt=Abstract&list_uids=1894388

- **Nocturnal biofeedback for nocturnal bruxism.**
  Author(s): Piccione A, Coates TJ, George JM, Rosenthal D, Karzmark P.

Source: Biofeedback Self Regul. 1982 December; 7(4): 405-19.
http://www.ncbi.nlm.nih.gov/entrez/query.fcgi?cmd=Retrieve&db=pubmed&dopt=A
bstract&list_uids=7165776

- **Nocturnal bruxism and temporomandibular disorders.**
  Author(s): Rugh JD, Harlan J.
  Source: Adv Neurol. 1988; 49: 329-41. Review.
  http://www.ncbi.nlm.nih.gov/entrez/query.fcgi?cmd=Retrieve&db=pubmed&dopt=A
  bstract&list_uids=3278546

- **Preauricular and head pain caused by bruxism.**
  Author(s): MONICA WS.
  Source: The Annals of Otology, Rhinology, and Laryngology. 1964 March; 73: 170-2.
  http://www.ncbi.nlm.nih.gov/entrez/query.fcgi?cmd=Retrieve&db=pubmed&dopt=A
  bstract&list_uids=14131353

- **Psychological approaches to the problem of bruxism.**
  Author(s): Romano JA.
  Source: J Bergen Cty Dent Soc. 1976 January; 42(4): 5-6. No Abstract Available.
  http://www.ncbi.nlm.nih.gov/entrez/query.fcgi?cmd=Retrieve&db=pubmed&dopt=A
  bstract&list_uids=1072062

- **Reduction of bruxism by contingent massage.**
  Author(s): Rudrud E, Halaszyn J.
  Source: Spec Care Dentist. 1981 May-June; 1(3): 122-4. No Abstract Available.
  http://www.ncbi.nlm.nih.gov/entrez/query.fcgi?cmd=Retrieve&db=pubmed&dopt=A
  bstract&list_uids=6940602

- **Self-monitoring in the treatment of diurnal bruxism.**
  Author(s): Rosen JC.
  Source: Journal of Behavior Therapy and Experimental Psychiatry. 1981 December;
  12(4): 347-50.
  http://www.ncbi.nlm.nih.gov/entrez/query.fcgi?cmd=Retrieve&db=pubmed&dopt=A
  bstract&list_uids=7199540

- **Suggestions for use of behavioral measures in treating bruxism.**
  Author(s): Cherasia M, Parks L.
  Source: Psychological Reports. 1986 June; 58(3): 719-22.
  http://www.ncbi.nlm.nih.gov/entrez/query.fcgi?cmd=Retrieve&db=pubmed&dopt=A
  bstract&list_uids=3726022

- **Suggestive hypnotherapy for nocturnal bruxism: a pilot study.**
  Author(s): Clarke JH, Reynolds PJ.
  Source: Am J Clin Hypn. 1991 April; 33(4): 248-53.
  http://www.ncbi.nlm.nih.gov/entrez/query.fcgi?cmd=Retrieve&db=pubmed&dopt=A
  bstract&list_uids=2024617

- **Temporal analysis of nocturnal bruxism during EMG feedback.**
  Author(s): Rugh JD, Johnson RW.

Source: J Periodontol. 1981 May; 52(5): 263-5.
http://www.ncbi.nlm.nih.gov/entrez/query.fcgi?cmd=Retrieve&db=pubmed&dopt=A
bstract&list_uids=6941011

- **Temporomandibular joint pain-dysfunction syndrome and bruxism: etiopathogenesis and treatment from a psychosomatic integrative viewpoint.**
  Author(s): Biondi M, Picardi A.
  Source: Psychotherapy and Psychosomatics. 1993; 59(2): 84-98. Review.
  http://www.ncbi.nlm.nih.gov/entrez/query.fcgi?cmd=Retrieve&db=pubmed&dopt=A
  bstract&list_uids=8332706

- **The application of audiostimulation and electromyographic biofeedback to bruxism and myofascial pain-dysfunction syndrome.**
  Author(s): Manns A, Miralles R, Adrian H.
  Source: Oral Surg Oral Med Oral Pathol. 1981 September; 52(3): 247-52. No Abstract Available.
  http://www.ncbi.nlm.nih.gov/entrez/query.fcgi?cmd=Retrieve&db=pubmed&dopt=A
  bstract&list_uids=6945531

- **The psychogenesis of bruxism.**
  Author(s): Walsh JP.
  Source: J Periodontol. 1965 September-October; 36(5): 417-20. No Abstract Available.
  http://www.ncbi.nlm.nih.gov/entrez/query.fcgi?cmd=Retrieve&db=pubmed&dopt=A
  bstract&list_uids=5212850

- **The psychological, physiological and hypnotic approach to bruxism in the treatment of periodontal disease.**
  Author(s): Goldberg G.
  Source: J Am Soc Psychosom Dent Med. 1973; 20(3): 75-91. No Abstract Available.
  http://www.ncbi.nlm.nih.gov/entrez/query.fcgi?cmd=Retrieve&db=pubmed&dopt=A
  bstract&list_uids=4525791

- **The reduction of bruxism using contingent EMG audible biofeedback: a case study.**
  Author(s): Feehan M, Marsh N.
  Source: Journal of Behavior Therapy and Experimental Psychiatry. 1989 June; 20(2): 179-83.
  http://www.ncbi.nlm.nih.gov/entrez/query.fcgi?cmd=Retrieve&db=pubmed&dopt=A
  bstract&list_uids=2584401

- **The treatment of bruxism--a review and analysis.**
  Author(s): Nadler SC.
  Source: The New York State Dental Journal. 1979 August-September; 45(7): 343-9. Review.
  http://www.ncbi.nlm.nih.gov/entrez/query.fcgi?cmd=Retrieve&db=pubmed&dopt=A
  bstract&list_uids=392359

- **The treatment of nocturnal bruxism using contingent EMG feedback with an arousal task.**
  Author(s): Clark GT, Beemstervoer P, Rugh JD.

Source: Behaviour Research and Therapy. 1981; 19(5): 451-5.
http://www.ncbi.nlm.nih.gov/entrez/query.fcgi?cmd=Retrieve&db=pubmed&dopt=A
bstract&list_uids=7316922

- **The use of biofeedback to control bruxism.**
  Author(s): Kardachi BJ, Clarke NG.
  Source: J Periodontol. 1977 October; 48(10): 639-42.
  http://www.ncbi.nlm.nih.gov/entrez/query.fcgi?cmd=Retrieve&db=pubmed&dopt=A
  bstract&list_uids=269244

- **Treatment approaches to bruxism.**
  Author(s): Thompson BA, Blount BW, Krumholz TS.
  Source: American Family Physician. 1994 May 15; 49(7): 1617-22. Review.
  http://www.ncbi.nlm.nih.gov/entrez/query.fcgi?cmd=Retrieve&db=pubmed&dopt=A
  bstract&list_uids=8184796

- **Treatment of nocturnal bruxism: a case study.**
  Author(s): Small MM.
  Source: Biological Psychology. 1978 April; 6(3): 235-6.
  http://www.ncbi.nlm.nih.gov/entrez/query.fcgi?cmd=Retrieve&db=pubmed&dopt=A
  bstract&list_uids=27254

- **Tryptophan supplementation for nocturnal bruxism: report of negative results.**
  Author(s): Etzel KR, Stockstill JW, Rugh JD, Fisher JG.
  Source: J Craniomandib Disord. 1991 Spring; 5(2): 115-20.
  http://www.ncbi.nlm.nih.gov/entrez/query.fcgi?cmd=Retrieve&db=pubmed&dopt=A
  bstract&list_uids=1812137

- **Understanding change: five-year follow-up of brief hypnotic treatment of chronic bruxism.**
  Author(s): LaCrosse MB.
  Source: Am J Clin Hypn. 1994 April; 36(4): 276-81.
  http://www.ncbi.nlm.nih.gov/entrez/query.fcgi?cmd=Retrieve&db=pubmed&dopt=A
  bstract&list_uids=8203355

- **Use of a portable electromyogram integrator and biofeedback unit in the treatment of chronic nocturnal bruxism.**
  Author(s): Hudzinski LG, Walters PJ.
  Source: The Journal of Prosthetic Dentistry. 1987 December; 58(6): 698-701.
  http://www.ncbi.nlm.nih.gov/entrez/query.fcgi?cmd=Retrieve&db=pubmed&dopt=A
  bstract&list_uids=3480357

- **Vectored upper cervical manipulation for chronic sleep bruxism, headache, and cervical spine pain in a child.**
  Author(s): Knutson GA.
  Source: Journal of Manipulative and Physiological Therapeutics. 2003 July-August; 26(6): E16.
  http://www.ncbi.nlm.nih.gov/entrez/query.fcgi?cmd=Retrieve&db=pubmed&dopt=A
  bstract&list_uids=12902973

Additional Web Resources

A number of additional Web sites offer encyclopedic information covering CAM and related topics. The following is a representative sample:

- Alternative Medicine Foundation, Inc.: **http://www.herbmed.org/**
- AOL: **http://search.aol.com/cat.adp?id=169&layer=&from=subcats**
- Chinese Medicine: **http://www.newcenturynutrition.com/**
- drkoop.com®: **http://www.drkoop.com/InteractiveMedicine/IndexC.html**
- Family Village: **http://www.familyvillage.wisc.edu/med_altn.htm**
- Google: **http://directory.google.com/Top/Health/Alternative/**
- Healthnotes: **http://www.healthnotes.com/**
- MedWebPlus: **http://medwebplus.com/subject/Alternative_and_Complementary_Medicine**
- Open Directory Project: **http://dmoz.org/Health/Alternative/**
- HealthGate: **http://www.tnp.com/**
- WebMD®Health: **http://my.webmd.com/drugs_and_herbs**
- WholeHealthMD.com: **http://www.wholehealthmd.com/reflib/0,1529,00.html**
- Yahoo.com: **http://dir.yahoo.com/Health/Alternative_Medicine/**

The following is a specific Web list relating to bruxism; please note that any particular subject below may indicate either a therapeutic use, or a contraindication (potential danger), and does not reflect an official recommendation:

- **General Overview**

    Temporomandibular Joint Dysfunction
    Source: Integrative Medicine Communications; www.drkoop.com

    TMJ
    Source: Integrative Medicine Communications; www.drkoop.com

General References

A good place to find general background information on CAM is the National Library of Medicine. It has prepared within the MEDLINEplus system an information topic page dedicated to complementary and alternative medicine. To access this page, go to the MEDLINEplus site at **http://www.nlm.nih.gov/medlineplus/alternativemedicine.html**. This Web site provides a general overview of various topics and can lead to a number of general sources.

CHAPTER 3. PATENTS ON BRUXISM

Overview

Patents can be physical innovations (e.g. chemicals, pharmaceuticals, medical equipment) or processes (e.g. treatments or diagnostic procedures). The United States Patent and Trademark Office defines a patent as a grant of a property right to the inventor, issued by the Patent and Trademark Office.[4] Patents, therefore, are intellectual property. For the United States, the term of a new patent is 20 years from the date when the patent application was filed. If the inventor wishes to receive economic benefits, it is likely that the invention will become commercially available within 20 years of the initial filing. It is important to understand, therefore, that an inventor's patent does not indicate that a product or service is or will be commercially available. The patent implies only that the inventor has "the right to exclude others from making, using, offering for sale, or selling" the invention in the United States. While this relates to U.S. patents, similar rules govern foreign patents.

In this chapter, we show you how to locate information on patents and their inventors. If you find a patent that is particularly interesting to you, contact the inventor or the assignee for further information. **IMPORTANT NOTE:** When following the search strategy described below, you may discover non-medical patents that use the generic term "bruxism" (or a synonym) in their titles. To accurately reflect the results that you might find while conducting research on bruxism, we have not necessarily excluded non-medical patents in this bibliography.

Patents on Bruxism

By performing a patent search focusing on bruxism, you can obtain information such as the title of the invention, the names of the inventor(s), the assignee(s) or the company that owns or controls the patent, a short abstract that summarizes the patent, and a few excerpts from the description of the patent. The abstract of a patent tends to be more technical in nature, while the description is often written for the public. Full patent descriptions contain much more information than is presented here (e.g. claims, references, figures, diagrams, etc.). We

---

[4]Adapted from the United States Patent and Trademark Office:
http://www.uspto.gov/web/offices/pac/doc/general/whatis.htm.

will tell you how to obtain this information later in the chapter. The following is an example of the type of information that you can expect to obtain from a patent search on bruxism:

- **Anti-bruxism device**

  Inventor(s): Lee, Jr.; Alexander Y. (1075 S. Jefferson St., Apt. 321, Arlington, VA 22204)

  Assignee(s): none reported

  Patent Number: 4,838,283

  Date filed: November 13, 1987

  Abstract: An apparatus and method for the control and prevention of bruxing (nocturnal teeth grinding) which comprises a sound generating means affixed to one area of the face of the user, a sound receiving means affixed to another area of the face, and an electronic control means to "read" signals from said sound receiver and to activate an alarm when bruxing occurs. Said apparatus utilizes the principle of bone conduction whereby the sonic vibrations from said second generator are transmitted to said sound receiver bottom when the jaw of the user is closed than when it is open. The alarm develops a conditioned reflex in the user such that after the first few alarms incident to bruxing the user does not awaken but merely reacts by relaxing the jaw when the alarm occurs.

  Excerpt(s): Bruxism is the condition of nocturnal **teeth grinding** which afflicts many people and which is widely considered to be a psychological stress reaction. The condition produces abnormal wear of the molar teeth of the afflicted person and is a source of annoyance and disturbance to anyone who sleeps in the near vicinity of such a person. Several devices have been patented which were designed to relieve the condition of **bruxism**. Among such devices are the Samelson inventions, U.S. Pat. Nos. 4,169,473 and 4,304,227. These inventions consist of molded devices designed to be inserted into the mouth of a person who experiences snoring and **bruxism** during sleep. The object of these inventions is to prevent nocturnal **teeth grinding** by means of an intervening physical barrier and to prevent snoring by means of forced nasal breathing. Another device, the Ober invention, U.S. Pat. No. 4,669,477 is an electronic instrument which operates by detecting electromyographic signal voltages from the mandibular musculature during bruxing. The device then imparts an electrical stimulation to the jaw of the bruxing person, which stimulation is intended to cause the jaw muscles to relax and allow the jaw to open. The Ober disclosure does not, however, reveal how said stimulation will selectively stimulate the particular muscle fibers that cause the jaw to open rather than resulting in the tonus of all the muscle fibers in the region of the stimulation.

  Web site: http://www.delphion.com/details?pn=US04838283__

- **Apparatus and method for preventing bruxism**

  Inventor(s): Ober; Stephen H. (Salt Lake City, UT)

  Assignee(s): Empi, Inc. (Fridley, MN)

  Patent Number: 4,669,477

  Date filed: May 20, 1985

  Abstract: Apparatus for producing an electrical stimulation signal adapted to be applied to a patient's jaw muscle, thereby causing the jaw to open and preventing **bruxism**. The apparatus includes electrodes positioned to sense an electromyographic (EMG) signal indicative of jaw muscle activity and jaw clenching. A control circuit produces a control signal when the EMG signal exceeds a threshold value indicative of a predetermined level of jaw muscle activity. Stimulator means produce the stimulation signal in the form of a pulse train when triggered by the control signal. The threshold value and intensity of the stimulation signal are adjustable.

Excerpt(s): The present invention relates to electrical neuromuscular stimulators. In particular, the present invention is a stimulator for preventing **bruxism**. Bruxism, the grinding or clenching of teeth during sleep, is a leading cause of temporal mandibular joint dysfunction and abnormal wearing of molar teeth. This affliction is believed to be caused by two phenomena. The first is maloclusion, the faulty closure of teeth. The second is psychological stress. As a learned behavior and an outlet from psychological stress, **bruxism** is exceedingly difficult to treat because it occurs during sleep when conscious activity and volitional control are non-existant. A common method of treating **bruxism** involves placing a splint between dental surfaces during sleep. While a device of this type will alleviate some of the effects of **bruxism,** it is of no help in preventing the underlying problem. The same can be said for many of the devices disclosed in the patent literature. The Samelson U.S. Pat. Nos. 4,169,473, and 4,304,227 disclose a device for treatment of snoring and **bruxism**. The device is molded for cooperation with the upper and lower dental surfaces and eliminates nocturnal **tooth grinding** when positioned within the mouth of the user.

Web site: http://www.delphion.com/details?pn=US04669477__

- **Apparatus and method for treating temporomadibular joint dysfunction and bruxism**

    Inventor(s): Anderson; Kent (4015 Creek View Ct., Rocklin, CA 95677)

    Assignee(s): none reported

    Patent Number: 4,976,618

    Date filed: May 30, 1989

    Abstract: The present invention provides an intraoral sensing device which generates a pressure change in cavities positioned between the upper and lower dental surfaces. This signal is used to provide a therapeutic apparatus and method for treatment of temporomandibular joint dysfunction and **bruxism**. An audible signal is generated to wake the patient from a nocturnal eqisode of abnormal jaw muscle activity. Control means are provided to establish a threshold value below which no audio signal is generated.

    Excerpt(s): This invention relates generally to apparatus and methods which are useful in the diagnosis and treatment of stress-related temporomandibular dysfunction and **bruxism**. More specifically, this invention relates to an intraoral device which can detect abnormal jaw muscle activity associated with these conditions by a gas or fluid pressure change in a flexible channel positioned between the posterior occlusal portions of the mouth. The mandible is connected to the cranium by the temporomandibular joints, located immediately in front of the ears. Rotation of the mandible about these joints is accomplished by the masticatory muscles, each of which extends from an opposite side of the mandible to a connecting point on the cranial bones. The masticatory muscles have an at rest position between their extended and contracted states. Under normal physiological conditions involving the outgrowth of a full complement of teeth, the mandibular portion of each temporomandibular joint will rest lightly in the cranial portion of the joint, and the muscles will be relaxed, or at rest. Masticatory muscle related stresses and/or pain can arise due to differences in occlusal pressures along the upper and lower dental arches. Temporomandibular joint dysfunction syndrome relates to occlusion-muscle incompatibility. Masticatory muscle accommodation is a key factor in the etiology of this syndrome. Psychological tension and stress can lead to temporomandibular joint dysfunction or **bruxism** in otherwise stable mouths with normal occlusion.

Web site: http://www.delphion.com/details?pn=US04976618__

- **Appliance adapted to fit many mouth and tooth sizes for orthodontic correction and other uses**

   Inventor(s): Bergersen; Earl O (Winnetka, IL)

   Assignee(s): Ortho-Tain, Inc. (Bayamon, PR)

   Patent Number: 5,876,199

   Date filed: August 28, 1997

   Abstract: An orthodontic appliance for assisting in properly positioning teeth within the mouth of an individual which is capable of fitting various mouth and tooth sizes. The appliance includes a labial-buccal flange, a lingual flange spaced from the labial-buccal flange, both of which define a generally U-shaped configuration in the occlusal view, and an isthmus interconnecting the two flanges. At least one tooth trough is defined between the labial-buccal flange and the lingual flange for receiving either an upper or a lower row of the individual's teeth. The appliance includes no individual tooth sockets but instead utilizes pressure applied by the labial-buccal flange, the lingual flange, and the relative angles and material thicknesses to properly position the teeth. The appliance is capable of fitting mouths and teeth of various sizes because it includes no individual tooth sockets. The appliance is also useful as a device for preventing sleep apnea, snoring and **bruxism** as well as an athletic mouth guard.

   Excerpt(s): The present invention relates to tooth positioning appliances, and in particular to a prefabricated appliance of one size which accommodates various mouth and tooth sizes and is useful as an orthodontic corrective device, an athletic mouthguard, a **bruxism** inhibitor, and a sleep apnea prevention device and snoring prevention device. There are many tooth malocclusion conditions which are correctable through orthodontic treatment. Some of these conditions include incisal spacing, overjet, overbite, incisal crowding, tooth rotation and improper jaw relations. Metal bands and wires are often used in the permanent dentition stage to provide the desired correction. Thermoplastic removable positioners or appliances are also available such as those disclosed in my prior U.S. Pat. Nos. 4,139,944; 4,919,612; 3,848,335; and 3,939,598. These removable appliances are typically provided with tooth sockets each for receiving therein one of the individual's teeth for guiding and directing the tooth into a proper occlusal position. Such appliances are therefore selected by measuring the individual's mouth and teeth and matching the appropriate sized appliance having the appropriate tooth socket sizes and spacing.

   Web site: http://www.delphion.com/details?pn=US05876199__

- **Bruxism biofeedback apparatus and method**

  Inventor(s): Burns; Clay (New York, NY), Devlin; Thomas E. (Somerville, MA), Ulrich; Karl T. (Narberth, PA), Weinstein; Lee (Arlington, MA)

  Assignee(s): BruxCare L.L.C. (Houston, TX)

  Patent Number: 6,117,092

  Date filed: November 23, 1998

  Abstract: A method and apparatus for the treatment of **bruxism** through biofeedback is disclosed. In one embodiment, the apparatus consists of electronics (M1) mounted in a light-weight headband (HB1) which may be worn comfortably by a user during sleep or while awake. Electrodes (E) within the headband pick up surface EMG voltage signals indicative of **bruxism,** and biofeedback is provided to the user through an earphone (SK).

  Excerpt(s): The invention relates generally to the fields of electromyographic monitoring and biofeedback, and more specifically to biofeedback devices and techniques for treating **bruxism.** Bruxism has generally been defined as the nonfunctional clenching, grinding, gritting, gnashing, and/or clicking of the teeth. **Bruxism** can occur while a person is awake or asleep. When the phenomenon occurs during sleep, it is called nocturnal **bruxism.** Even when it occurs during waking hours, the bruxer is often not conscious of the activity. Biting force exerted during **bruxism** often significantly exceeds peak biting force exerted during normal chewing. Biting forces exceeding 700 pounds have been measured during bruxing events. Chronic **bruxism** may result in musculoskeletal pain, headaches, and damage to the teeth and/or the temporomandibular joint. The primary treatment for nocturnal **bruxism** is the use of intra-oral occlusal splints or "mouth guards," which are generally semi-rigid plastic covers for the upper or lower teeth. Occlusal splints are generally fabricated for a specific individual from an impression taken of the individual's teeth. While some studies have shown that the wearing of an occlusal splint may reduce bruxing event duration and intensity, the large replacement market for "chewed up" occlusal splints attests to the role of the splint primarily to protect teeth from damage, rather than as a cure for **bruxism.** Even as a symptomatic treatment, occlusal splints often only protect the teeth themselves, while the user may still suffer musculoskeletal pain and possible damage to the temporomandibular joint.

  Web site: http://www.delphion.com/details?pn=US06117092__

- **Bruxism method and apparatus using electrical signals**

  Inventor(s): Perry, Jr.; John D. (242 Old Eagle School Rd., Strafford, PA 19087)

  Assignee(s): none reported

  Patent Number: 4,934,378

  Date filed: March 31, 1989

  Abstract: The invention measures the electrical signals at the microvolt level emitted from the masseteric (jaw) muscle when **bruxism** occurs. The apparatus detects electrical signal impulses from electrodes on a transducer probe located within one of the patient's ear channels and transmits the detected signals to an amplifier. in one embodiment, a circuit converts the signal information into an audible tone. The tone provides the immediate knowledge of the **bruxism** which leads to controlling of the action. The apparatus may be worn inconspicuously during the day and without discomfort while asleep for sleep interruption feedback.

Excerpt(s): The present invention relates to the dental methods and apparatus for the treatment of **bruxism,** i.e., the grinding of teeth. **Bruxism** is the abnormal excessive and non-functional nocturnal or subconscious grinding of teeth. Clinically significant **bruxism** may ruin the teeth and may indicate, or lead to, temporomandibular Joint Dysfunction (TMJ) or Myofascical Pain Dysfunction (MPD). In TMJ the muscles used for chewing and the joints of the jaw fail to work in conjunction. Due to emotional stress, some people clench their teeth so hard that they jolt their jaw out of its natural position, resulting in TMJ. The misalignment of the temporomandibular joint (jaw joint) causes muscle spasms, resulting in pain in front of the ear and in the head. Thee pain may also spread to the neck, shoulders and back. The initials MPD have been used to refer to similar terms: "myofascial", "myofacial", "masticatory" or "mandibular" pain dysfunction, see Schwartz, M. Biofeedback: A Practitioner's Guide, Ch 16, pgs. 288-307 (1987).

Web site: http://www.delphion.com/details?pn=US04934378__

- **Dental appliance for alleviating snoring and protecting teeth from bruxism**

Inventor(s): Gottehrer; Neil R. (202 Clwyd Rd., Bala Cynwyd, PA 19004), Misch; Carl Erwin (410 Claremount, Dearborn, MI 48124), Singer; Gary H. (1717 W. Chester Pike, Havertown, PA 19083)

Assignee(s): none reported

Patent Number: 5,823,193

Date filed: January 27, 1997

Abstract: A single dental appliance that both alleviates snoring and protects teeth from **bruxism.** The appliance (10) has an upper section (12) which is mounted on the upper jaw. Opposing the upper section (12) is a lower section (14) which is mounted on the lower jaw. Both the upper and lower section have an anterior region (16, 18) and two posterior regions (20, 22; 24, 26). A hard outer shell (32, 34) secures in a soft inner liner (28, 30) which conforms with the teeth and cushions the jaw against impact forces. The hard outer shell (32, 34) serves to protect the teeth against grinding. The combination of the liner and the shell distribute forces associated with grinding.

Excerpt(s): This invention relates to a single dental appliance which both protects teeth from **bruxism** and alleviates snoring. Bruxism is the vertical and horizontal, non-functional grinding of teeth. The forces involved often exceed the normal physiologic masticatory loads (up to 1,000 psi). **Bruxism** may adversely affect teeth, muscles and joints, or all three. Such adverse effects may occur while the patient is awake or asleep. Use of a bite guard is helpful for many **bruxism** patients. A bite guard, in one form, resembles a semi-transparent mouth guard that a boxer or football player might wear to protect his teeth. The guard is placed over the teeth to protect them from grinding.

Web site: http://www.delphion.com/details?pn=US05823193__

- **Dental applicance for treating bruxism**

Inventor(s): Schaefer, deceased; Donald W. (late of Madison, WI), Siedband; Melvin P. (Madison, WI)

Assignee(s): Schaefer Partnership (Eau Claire, WI)

Patent Number: 5,490,520

Date filed: September 27, 1993

Abstract: A dental appliance for treating **bruxism** is provided which, according to one aspect of the invention, has a mouthpiece containing an electric source, electrodes, and circuitry connecting the source to the electrodes, and circuitry connecting the source to the electrodes. The electrodes are disposed to contact an interior surface of the wearer's mouth to conduct electric stimuli to the mouth. Included in the electronic circuitry, are sensors which trigger the flow of electric current from the source to the electrodes when squeezed together by the wearer's teeth.

Excerpt(s): This invention relates to dental appliances, particularly to mouthpieces used to treat bruxing. Many people, for reasons not clearly understood, grind their teeth at night while sleeping. The usual complaints related by this group of people are soreness in joints, facial muscles, and neck muscles, headaches, clicking of the jaw, earaches, etc. Most of these people seek help from their dentist or physician who cite headache disorders, cranial neuralgia and facial pain as the most common symptoms. This grinding of the teeth is called bruxing. Commonly, the grinding of the teeth takes place during the night and the condition is referred to as nocturnal **bruxism.** Such clenching and grinding of the teeth can also lead to the onset of temporomandibular joint syndrome or temporomandibular disfunction referred to as TMJ syndrome or TMD. In spite of the fact that there has been an explosion of interest and research regarding **bruxism** and TMJ disorders in the past ten years, the most common treatment continues to be the "night splint" usually prescribed by dentists. A night splint is a plastic dental appliance made from a model of the patient's teeth and is designed to fit firmly on either the upper or lower teeth. The night splint is usually fitted to the upper teeth and is somewhat similar to a boxer's mouthpiece.

Web site: http://www.delphion.com/details?pn=US05490520__

- **Dental protector against bruxism**

Inventor(s): Yoshida; Nobutaka (9-18, Nipponbashi 2-chome, Chuo-ku, Osaka-shi, Osaka 542-0073, JP)

Assignee(s): none reported

Patent Number: 6,302,110

Date filed: May 25, 1999

Abstract: The invention has for its object to provide a dental protector against **bruxism** adapted to protect the teeth from clenching, insure stability during wear, and applicable to many persons. The dental protector comprises a protective part (2) configured generally in the form of the letter U in conformity with the dental arc and adapted to cover the occlusal faces of the teeth and an engaging part (3) contiguous to the inner circumference of the protective part and adapted to cover the posterior surfaces of the teeth, the lower stratum (2y) of the protective part, which is to contact with the teeth, and the engaging part being formed from a thermoplastic resin having a softening temperature lower than the boiling temperature of water and the upper stratum (2x) of the protective part which is flat being formed from a material which does not soften at the above softening temperature.

Excerpt(s): This invention relates to a dental protector for prevention of the nuisance associated with **bruxism,** i.e. clenching of the teeth, which is mounted on the teeth at bedtime. While some persons grind their teeth unconsciously during sleep, this phenomenon known as **bruxism** produces noises offensive to the ear, causing a great nuisance to their roommates in many cases. Moreover, as **bruxism** becomes severe, it imposes so great a burden on one's own teeth that the teeth are sometimes worn or injured. Therefore, it is common practice that the dentist takes an impression of the oral cavity to fabricate a plaster cast and causes a filled acrylic resin material to polymerize in suit to construct a dental protector conforming to the upper and lower teeth, and let the patient wear the device.

Web site: http://www.delphion.com/details?pn=US06302110__

- **Device for preventing bruxism**

Inventor(s): Burger; Michael A. (Pasqualinistraat S, 5622 AW Eindhoven, NL), Martens; Rigobertus W. (Schweitzerlaan 2S, 5644 DL Eindhoven, NL)

Assignee(s): none reported

Patent Number: 5,553,626

Date filed: February 9, 1995

Abstract: An anti **bruxism** device for stopping or at least diminishing **bruxism** comprises a splint adapted to be secured to a tooth of a user, and a biofeedback system mounted on the splint. The biofeedback system includes a detector for detecting **bruxism,** and a stimulation device for stimulating the user responsive to detection of **bruxism** by the detector. The stimulation produced by the stimulation device causes the user to stop bruxating. **Bruxism** is a function that could damage teeth and molars, and may affect the neuro-muscular system in a negative way, and could cause, for example, headaches.

Excerpt(s): The invention concerns an anti-bruxism device. **Bruxism** is a conscious or subconscious parafunction that takes place during the day and/or at night, and consists of a static and/or dynamic contact between the chewing levels of the mandibular and upper jaw. The purpose of the invention is to develop a device that stops **bruxism** and raises the hurtful accesories. The device consists of an already used splint (synthetic resin) as carrier for a special biofeedback system. A splint is a synthetic resin modelled plate most frequently worn on the teeth of the upper jaw. The biofeedback system detects **bruxism,** transponds a signal which diminishes, and finally stops **bruxism.** This device can also be used for preventive means; that is to say with patients grinding their teeth who don't yet suffer the consequences.

Web site: http://www.delphion.com/details?pn=US05553626__

- **Device for sensing and treating bruxism**

  Inventor(s): Matz; Warren W. (882 U.S. Highway 1, Juno Beach, FL 33408)

  Assignee(s): none reported

  Patent Number: 5,586,562

  Date filed: July 14, 1995

  Abstract: The instant invention is a device and method for treatment of **bruxism,** snoring, and sleep apnea based upon an inconspicuously placed tooth guard which, in the preferred embodiment, includes a pressure sensitive surface which is electrically coupled to an alarm mechanism. The alarm mechanism is activated when the contact area is compressed and may be constructed of sensitive materials so as to detect vibrations indicative of snoring. The device attaches to release clips bonded to the side of a tooth with a sensing area positioned between the teeth so as to indicate **bruxism** is occurring. The alarm mechanism will provide a resonant frequency capable of making a sound or providing a vibration indicating to the individual that **bruxism** is occurring. A timer mechanism can be used to delay operation of the alarm. Alternatively, the timer mechanism can be made operational wherein the lack of circuit contact will cause alarm so as to indicated sleep apnea. An alternative embodiment of the invention provides a tooth guard as part of the **bruxism** treatment wherein once the alarm mechanism has broken the habit of **bruxism,** the guard reinforces anti-bruxism without the alarm function.

  Excerpt(s): This invention relates to **bruxism** and, more particularly, to a device for sensing and treating **bruxism.** Teeth are hard calcified structures attached to the upper and lower jaws of a human. Serving major functions such as chewing as well as providing for the formation of certain sounds by acting as a brace for the tongue, teeth can be divided into three general types: the incisors, the cuspids, and the molars. The incisors, or front teeth are spade shaped which facilitate in the cutting of food. Central and lateral incisors are positioned in each quarter of the mouth followed by three cuspid teeth used in ripping of food. Two teeth in back of the cuspids are called the bi-cuspids each which have a cusp and are followed by first, second and third molars having a relatively flat chewing surface which permits the grinding or milling of food.

  Web site: http://www.delphion.com/details?pn=US05586562__

- **Device for treatment of snoring, bruxism or for avoidance of sleep apnea**

  Inventor(s): Samelson; Charles F. (5712 S. Kenwood, Chicago, IL 60637)

  Assignee(s): none reported

  Patent Number: 4,304,227

  Date filed: August 27, 1979

  Abstract: A device is provided for positioning within the mouth of a user for preventing snoring and nocturnal **tooth grinding.** The device is an integrally molded body. The device provides dental engaging portions and a rearwardly-opening central socket for cooperating with the forward portion of the user's tongue in a manner to draw the tongue forwardly so as to increase the unobstructed dimension of the nasal breathing passage. When operatively positioned within the mouth, some of the user's upper and lower teeth will enter into recesses provided by the device. The device substantially eliminates oral breathing. The tongue will be held in the socket by a negative pressure developed in the socket. When the tongue is held, it draws the body of the tongue forwardly of its usual restive position behind the lower teeth and adjacent the soft palate, the uvula and the posterior pharyngeal wall, thereby increasing the dimension of the air flow passage through the naso-pharynx to facilitate nasal breathing. The device's engagement with at least portions of one of the user's dental arches operates to eliminate nocturnal tooth-grinding.

Excerpt(s): This invention relates to an anti-snore and anti-tooth-grinding device, and more particularly, to a device for selective insertion within the mouth of a user so as to obstruct the oral flow of air past the lips of the user, and to increase the size of the air passageway through the oro- and naso-pharynx, and which may also be provided with means for immobilizing jaw movement. Snoring is caused by the relaxation of body tissue in the lingual compartment, the tissue including the tongue, the pharyngeal folds, the soft palate, the muscularis uvulae and the palate-pharyngeal arch. During normal waking hours, muscle tone in most individuals unconsciously maintains the above structures in adequate spacial relationships so as not to interfere with the free passage of air therepast. However, with increasing age, and during periods of unconsciousness, some muscle tone is lost, thereby allowing one or more of the tongue, the pharyngeal folds, the soft palate, the uvulae and the posterior pharyngeal wall to vibrate as tidal air flows therepast. While the act of snoring is socially discomfitting to other persons who hear the snores, and especially annoying to a spouse attempting to sleep, it can also cause harmful complications to the snorer, such as disturbed rest, excessive drying of the oro- and naso-pharyngeal mucous membranes with consequent injury to the throat, middle and inner ear, susceptibility to infection, vertigo and impaired hearing. Of equal importance is the fact that people who snore are not making use of the physiologically beneficial aspects of nasal breathing. The anatomical nasal structures (such as the turbinates, mucous membranes, etc.) provide moistening and cleansing functions during sleep.

Web site: http://www.delphion.com/details?pn=US04304227__

- **Measurement device for quantifying the severity of bruxism**

Inventor(s): Burns; Clay A. (New York, NY), McDonald; K. Alex (Houston, TX), Ulrich; Karl T. (Narberth, PA), Weinstein; Lee (Somerville, MA)

Assignee(s): BruxCare, L.L.C. (Austin, TX)

Patent Number: 5,911,576

Date filed: January 13, 1998

Abstract: A **bruxism** monitoring device comprising a thin shell formed to the shape of and elastically retained to one or more teeth, said shell further comprising: a plurality of layers having mutually distinguishable colors, each color distinguishable from the colors of adjacent layers; and a material thickness that is greater anteriorly than posteriorly. The outer layer of the shell, when worn away by grinding action, reveals an inner layer. The regions of wear may be analyzed to determine the extent of the bruxing activity.

Excerpt(s): This invention relates to **bruxism** measurement devices and more particularly to an intraoral appliance for quantifying the extent of wear due to the grinding action of teeth. Bruxism has generally been defined as the nonfunctional clenching, grinding, gritting, gnashing, and clicking of the teeth. **Bruxism** can occur while a person is awake or asleep. When the phenomenon occurs during sleep, it is called nocturnal **bruxism.** Even when it occurs during waking hours, the bruxist is often not conscious of the activity. Biting force exerted during **bruxism** often significantly exceeds peak biting force exerted during normal chewing. Biting forces exceeding 700 pounds have been measured during bruxing events. Chronic **bruxism** may result in musculoskeletal pain, headaches, and damage to the teeth and/or the temporomandibular joint. The symptoms of **bruxism** include: clicking or grinding noises detected by a sleeping partner, wear facets on a bruxist's tooth surfaces, jaw pain, headaches, damage to teeth or dental work, and over development of the jaw muscles. When **bruxism** is severe, it may be accurately diagnosed by the presence of jaw pain and over development of the jaw muscles. When **bruxism** is less severe, it may be difficult to diagnose. For example, wear facets are often detected by a dentist during a dental examination, but may have resulted from bruxing during a previous period of the patient's life. Because nocturnal **bruxism** is a subconscious activity, bruxists may not be aware of their bruxing and may not believe that they brux even when presented with strong circumstantial evidence.

Web site: http://www.delphion.com/details?pn=US05911576__

- **Method and apparatus for sensing and treating bruxism**

Inventor(s): Burman; Dennis A. (449 Curie Dr., San Jose, CA 95123), Gallia; Louis J. (2259 Swarthmore St., Sacramento, CA 95825), Nordlander; Jeffrey Y. (1020 40th St., Sacramento, CA 95819)

Assignee(s): Gallia; Louis J. (Sacramento, CA), Nordlander; Jeffrey Y. (Sacramento, CA)

Patent Number: 5,078,153

Date filed: September 17, 1990

Abstract: An intraoral acrylic splint having incorporated into the interior of the splint a strip of piezoelectric film which emits a small electrical current when deformed by the compression of the teeth. The piezoelectric film is connected by conductors to a small battery powered radio transmitter contained in the splint. The transmitter generates and broadcasts a radio frequency signal when current is received from the piezoelectric film. The radio frequency signal is received by a remote receiver unit. The receiver unit emits an audible alarm upon receiving a signal from the radio transmitter of the splint. The audible alarm alerts the patient of his action, allowing him to consciously resist bruxing.

Excerpt(s): This invention relates to methods and devices used to detect and control **bruxism.** The habit of a person grinding his teeth is especially difficult to treat since the action occurs most often when the person is asleep and unaware of the occurrence. This habit may be so unconscious it can also occur during waking hours without the person being aware of it. If left untreated, the habit may lead to permanent deterioration of the teeth, displacement of internal temporomandibular structures, and pain during mastication. A major cause of bruxing appears to be emotional or psychological stress which triggers an innate physiologic response of clenching or grinding the teeth. The nocturnal occurrence and unconsciousness of the response make the problem extremely difficult to treat. Awareness of each episode of **bruxism** can enable the person to gain control of the activity and thereby reduce or eliminate the symptoms.

Web site: http://www.delphion.com/details?pn=US05078153__

- **Multifunctional behavioral modification device for snoring, bruxism, and apnea**

  Inventor(s): Crossley; Robert B. (6600 Elm Creek No. 152, Austin, TX 78744)

  Assignee(s): none reported

  Patent Number: 4,715,367

  Date filed: September 15, 1986

  Abstract: A multifunctional behavioral modification device to diagnose, treat and monitor treatment for snoring, **bruxism,** or sleep apnea. Treatment consists of regulatable aversive shock, automatically occurring with each audible sound from snoring until snoring ceases or continuously but pulsatingly administered from clenching or grinding of teeth until the action ceases or continuously but pulsatingly administered from sleep apnea until breathing restarts. The placement of electrodes for administering the regulatable aversive shock is such so as to actuate a motor nerve thereby allowing use of a shock so mild as not to awaken a sleeper but sufficient to condition against the adverse behavior being sensed.

  Excerpt(s): This invention comprises a basic device used with different sensing means to detect and treat snoring, **bruxism** or sleep apnea. Bruxism has been defined as the non-purposeful grinding or clenching of teeth. This results in excessive teeth wear and in some cases loosening and loss of teeth. Other physical problems such as headaches and deterioration of jawbone joint also may occur. Of course the excessive grinding noise may also be deleterious to relationships with others as well. Sleep apnea is a cessation of breathing during sleep that results in the person awakening for no reason he or she may be conscious of or of partial awakening or sleeping fitfully. Sleep apnea has been difficult to diagnose in a simple fashion. One of the objects of this invention is to allow simple diagnosis of sleep apnea.

  Web site: http://www.delphion.com/details?pn=US04715367__

- **Systems for modifying behavioral disorders**

  Inventor(s): Morris; Donald E. (44 Marguerita Rd., Kensington, CA 94707)

  Assignee(s): none reported

  Patent Number: 6,093,158

  Date filed: May 14, 1998

  Abstract: A system is provided for monitoring an undesired behavioral disorder such as **bruxism,** jaw clenching, or snoring. A processor correlates the monitored behavior with the onset of the undesired disorder. Since behavior of this type is typically subconscious, the sensor is preferably coupled to a warning device to alert the patient when he or she is performing the undesired behavior. Typically the warning device causes the patient to experience an unpleasant sensation, thus promoting the discontinuance of the behavior. In one embodiment the system determines which stimuli is most effective and therefore best suited for an individual patient. The system may further include means to record the monitored data related to the undesired behavioral disorders. This feature allows the patient to receive data related to the rate, duration, intensity, and time of day that the unconscious behavior occurred thus allowing the patient to correlate the undesired behavior with outside factors.

  Excerpt(s): The present invention relates to a system and method for the treatment of sleeping disorders such as **bruxism,** jaw clenching, and snoring. **Bruxism** is the abnormal excessive and non-functional nocturnal or subconscious grinding of teeth which may or may not be associated with jaw clenching. Snoring is typically related to the manner of breathing (i.e., through the mouth as opposed to through the nose), the sleeping position (i.e., on the back versus on the side), or both. At a minimum, **bruxism** and jaw clenching will typically result in excessive tooth wear and periodontal problems. Unfortunately in many cases this clenching or bruxing action not only damages the teeth themselves, but also the supporting structure of the teeth including both the hard bony material and the soft tissue. As a result, in more extreme cases these disorders lead to TMJ, jaw displacement, stiff neck, and severe headaches. Research on **bruxism** has shown that **bruxism** is linked with stress. Although not everyone who bruxes is under stress, it has been shown that some people grind their teeth more after a tense day, or in the anticipation of stress. As stress, or the perception of stress occurs, **bruxism** is likely to occur. Snoring, unlike **bruxism,** may or may not be related to stress. Typically snoring is simply a consequence of how a person breathes while they sleep or the position in which they sleep. Often snoring is symptomatic of another problem, such as an allergy, which affects the way in which a person breathes. Therefore once a solution is found to the root problem, the snoring problem may disappear. Unfortunately not all snoring is related to such a solvable root problem.

Web site: http://www.delphion.com/details?pn=US06093158__

- **Taste-based approach to the prevention of teeth clenching and grinding**

  Inventor(s): Nissani; Moti (24281 Cloverlawn, Oak Park, MI 48237)

  Assignee(s): none reported

  Patent Number: 6,164,278

  Date filed: February 25, 1999

  Abstract: A new biofeedback modality for the treatment of **bruxism.** A mildly aversive, safe, liquid is inserted into, and sealed in, small, bilaterally-sleeved, polyethylene capsules. Two capsules are attached to a specially-constructed dental appliance which comfortably and securely places them between the lower and upper teeth. The appliance and capsules are worn at night or at other times when **bruxism** is suspected to occur. Whenever a sleeping or an awake patient attempts to brux, the capsules rupture and the liquid is released into the mouth. The liquid then draws the patient's conscious attention to, and forestalls, any attempt of teeth clenching or grinding. Variations of the method and device can be used to diagnose **bruxism** and to sustainably release medications and odor-masking substances into the mouth,.

  Excerpt(s): The present invention relates chiefly to teeth clenching and grinding and, more specifically, to a method and devices for treating, diagnosing, and preventing **bruxism.** Bruxism can be defined as excessive grinding or clenching of teeth. This behavioral pattern is often unconscious and involuntary, and can take place while the patient is asleep or awake. In any event, and regardless of the exact number, it is inarguably the case that **bruxism** is a widespread behavioral pattern which adversely affects a significant fraction of the world's population. Thus, there is an urgent need for the development of effective therapies for treating this condition--any advance in this field will help improve the quality of life of millions.

  Web site: http://www.delphion.com/details?pn=US06164278__

- **Treatment of bruxism**

Inventor(s): Friedman; Mark (5 Forest Ct., Larchmont, NY 10538)

Assignee(s): none reported

Patent Number: 6,632,843

Date filed: February 1, 2000

Abstract: This invention relates to the use of a composition for local percutaneous delivery of a drug such as a muscle relaxant, more particularly cyclobenzaprine in an organogel cream. The composition is applied by the patient directly to the skin over accessible muscles of mastication i.e., masseter and temporalis. The composition is rapidly absorbed through the skin to provide control of harmful habits such as **bruxism** and tooth clenching. The composition can also be applied to the skin overlying these muscles to control muscle hyperactivity (spasm) and/or trigger points, from other causes. The composition can be formulated to include another active agent such as a non-steroidal anti-inflammatory, for example ketoprofen. The advantage of topical administration versus systemic include use of lower doses of drug, delivery of the drug to the desired site, avoidance of the gastrointestinal tract and hepatic first-pass biotransformation and metabolism, and elimination of many of the side effects of the drug normally associated with systemic administration.

Excerpt(s): This invention relates to the use of a composition for the local percutaneous delivery of at least one pharmaceutically active agent formulated in a lecithin organogel cream. In the preferred embodiment of the invention, the composition is formulated with the muscle relaxant, cyclobenzaprine. The composition is applied by the patient, directly to the skin, over accessible muscles of mastication (masseter and temporal is). Such a composition is rapidly absorbed through the skin to provide control of muscle tension and relief from pain resulting from **bruxism (tooth grinding)** and tooth clenching (isometric muscle contraction). Similarly a composition can be formulated comprising an additional pharmaceutically active agent such as a non-steroidal anti-inflammatory drug such as ketoprofen or other similarly active agent. Other pharmacologically active substances can also be added, for example an anti-anxiety compound such as diazepam. Bruxism (tooth grinding when not masticating or swallowing) and tooth clenching, (that is isometric muscle contraction with the teeth in contact) common of the functional jaw disturbances. The isometric contraction produced during clenching is even more tiring to the muscles than the isotonic contraction produced during **bruxism.** However, bruxing forces are still considerable. The volume of the sound produced during grinding is considerable and is difficult to simulate voluntarily. This excitation of the jaw closing muscles appears to serve as a tension-relieving mechanism. Some individuals are more susceptible to environmental stress, and respond by increased jaw muscle tension, either at night of with day time clenching. It has been postulated that the protective mechanism in these individuals has been dulled down. Experimental evidence has shown that in addition to discomfort, damage accompanies such muscular hyperactivity.

Web site: http://www.delphion.com/details?pn=US06632843__

Patent Applications on Bruxism

As of December 2000, U.S. patent applications are open to public viewing.[5] Applications are patent requests which have yet to be granted. (The process to achieve a patent can take several years.) The following patent applications have been filed since December 2000 relating to bruxism:

- **Apparatus for treating bruxism**

  Inventor(s): Yerushalmy, Israel; (Tel Aviv, IL)

  Correspondence: Dekel Patent LTD.; Beit Harofim; Room 27; 18 Menuha Venahala Street; Rehovot; IL

  Patent Application Number: 20030125661

  Date filed: January 3, 2002

  Abstract: Apparatus for the treatment of **bruxism**, including a biosensor adapted to sense a phenomenon associated with a bruxing event, and a relaxation stimulator in communication with the biosensor and adapted to provide a relaxation stimulus to relax at least one of an obruxism muscle and an obruxism nerve.

  Excerpt(s): The present invention relates generally to apparatus for treating **bruxism**. Bruxism has generally been defined as nonfunctional clenching, grinding, gritting, gnashing, and/or clicking of the teeth. **Bruxism** may occur while a person is awake or asleep. When the phenomenon occurs during sleep, it is called nocturnal **bruxism**. Even when it occurs during waking hours, the bruxer is often not conscious of the activity. Biting force exerted during **bruxism** often significantly exceeds peak biting force exerted during normal chewing. Chronic **bruxism** may result in musculoskeletal pain, headaches, and damage to the teeth and/or the temporomandibular joint. **Bruxism** has been connected with temporomandibular disorders (TMD) or temporomandibular joint (TMJ) syndrome. One of the known treatments in the prior art for nocturnal **bruxism** is the use of intra-oral occlusal splints or "mouth guards," which are generally semi-rigid plastic covers for the upper or lower teeth. Occlusal splints are generally fabricated for a specific individual from an impression taken of the individual's teeth. However, the occlusal splints often only protect the teeth themselves, while the user may still suffer musculoskeletal pain and possible damage to the temporomandibular joint. Moreover, occlusal splints present numerous inconveniences to the user. They may require frequent cleaning, may be difficult to clean, may require periodic replacement, may inhibit speech, and may be frequently lost.

  Web site: http://appft1.uspto.gov/netahtml/PTO/search-bool.html

- **Bruxism appliance and method of forming**

  Inventor(s): Zuk, Michael Yar; (Red Deer, CA)

  Correspondence: Borden Ladner Gervais, Llp; 1000 - 60 Queen Street; Ottawa; ON; K1p 5y7; CA

  Patent Application Number: 20010017136

  Date filed: January 12, 2001

---

[5] This has been a common practice outside the United States prior to December 2000.

Abstract: A **bruxism** appliance and a method of forming a **bruxism** appliance is described for providing a patient and a dentist with a visual indication of the degree of **bruxism** by the patient. The invention teaches the application of an abradable composition to the nonretaining/opposing dentition contacting surfaces of the appliance in order that specific wear patterns can be observed on the appliance following use by a patient.

Excerpt(s): Bruxism or grinding of the teeth is defined as rhythmic or spasmodic grinding of the teeth in other than chewing movements of the mandible, especially such movements performed during sleep. Dental malocclusion and tension-release factors are the usual inciting causes (Dorland's Illustrated Medical Dictionary,.sub.26th edition, W. B. Saunders Co.). It is a significant dental problem afflicting upwards of 30% of the population. As **bruxism** normally occurs at night and damage to the teeth from **bruxism** occurs slowly, most patients are unaware of the problem and only notice the damage to their teeth after significant wear has occurred. If left untreated **bruxism** will slowly result in severe wear of the dentition, cracks and fractures in the teeth and may result in premature tooth loss. The canine teeth are designed to be protective of the rest of the dentition by their large crown, root morphology and position. The reduction of the protective length of these teeth is commonly the first visible sign that **bruxism** has occurred. Large well developed masseter muscles are also a feature of severe bruxers. Apart from these indications, bruxers do not often exhibit symptoms such as pain and, as such, it is often difficult for a dentist to convince a patient that a significant problem exists, let alone suggest an appropriate method for prevention. In treating **bruxism,** most patients will often not respond to various forms of treatment such as bite or occlusal adjustments and orthodontics. Therefore, as they are unable to consciously prevent the damaging activity from occurring, a **bruxism** appliance, which forms a physical and softer barrier to grinding teeth, is often the only form of treatment that prevents further damage from occurring.

Web site: http://appft1.uspto.gov/netahtml/PTO/search-bool.html

Keeping Current

In order to stay informed about patents and patent applications dealing with bruxism, you can access the U.S. Patent Office archive via the Internet at the following Web address: **http://www.uspto.gov/patft/index.html**. You will see two broad options: (1) Issued Patent, and (2) Published Applications. To see a list of issued patents, perform the following steps: Under "Issued Patents," click "Quick Search." Then, type "bruxism" (or synonyms) into the "Term 1" box. After clicking on the search button, scroll down to see the various patents which have been granted to date on bruxism.

You can also use this procedure to view pending patent applications concerning bruxism. Simply go back to **http://www.uspto.gov/patft/index.html**. Select "Quick Search" under "Published Applications." Then proceed with the steps listed above.

CHAPTER 4. BOOKS ON BRUXISM

Overview

This chapter provides bibliographic book references relating to bruxism. In addition to online booksellers such as **www.amazon.com** and **www.bn.com**, excellent sources for book titles on bruxism include the Combined Health Information Database and the National Library of Medicine. Your local medical library also may have these titles available for loan.

Book Summaries: Federal Agencies

The Combined Health Information Database collects various book abstracts from a variety of healthcare institutions and federal agencies. To access these summaries, go directly to the following hyperlink: **http://chid.nih.gov/detail/detail.html**. You will need to use the "Detailed Search" option. To find book summaries, use the drop boxes at the bottom of the search page where "You may refine your search by." Select the dates and language you prefer. For the format option, select "Monograph/Book." Now type "bruxism" (or synonyms) into the "For these words:" box. You should check back periodically with this database which is updated every three months. The following is a typical result when searching for books on bruxism:

- **Instructions for Patients. 5th ed**

  Source: Orlando, FL: W.B. Saunders Company. 1994. 598 p.

  Contact: Available from W.B. Saunders Company. Order Fulfillment, 6277 Sea Harbor Drive, Orlando, FL 32887-4430. (800) 545-2522 (individuals) or (800) 782-4479 (schools); Fax (800) 874-6418 or (407) 352-3445; http://www.wbsaunders.com. PRICE: $52.00 (English); $49.95 (Spanish); plus shipping and handling. ISBN: 0721649300 (English); 0721669972 (Spanish).

  Summary: This book is a compilation of instructions for patients, published in paperback format. The fact sheets each provide information in three sections: basic information, including a description of the condition, frequent signs and symptoms, causes, risk factors, preventive measures, expected outcome, and possible complications; treatment, including general measures, medication, activity guidelines, and diet; and when to contact one's health care provider. Fact sheets are available on oral health topics including: herpangina, leukoplakia, lichen planus, salivary gland infection, benign mouth or tongue tumors, oral cancer, periodontitis, salivary gland tumors, Sjogren's syndrome, stomatitis, teething, temporomandibular joint syndrome (TMJ), oral candidiasis (thrush), thumbsucking, glossitis (tongue inflammation), **bruxism** (tooth grinding), necrotizing ulcerative gingivitis (trench mouth), and trigeminal neuralgia (tic douloureux). The fact sheets are designed to be photocopied and distributed to patients as a reinforcement of oral instructions and as a teaching tool.

- **Physical Therapy in Craniomandibular Disorders**

Source: Carol Stream, IL: Quintessence Publishing Company, Inc. 1992. 80 p.

Contact: Available from Quintessence Publishing Company, Inc. 551 North Kimberly Drive, Carol Stream, IL 60188-1881. (800) 621-0387 or (630) 682-3223; Fax (630) 682-3288; E-mail: quintpub@aol.com; http://www.quintpub.com. PRICE: $36.00 plus shipping and handling. ISBN: 0867151927.

Summary: This book on physical therapy (PT) in craniomandibular disorders (CMD) outlines practical strategies for physical therapists and dentists who strive to provide treatment using a team approach. The authors hope to help standardize the management of CMD, and familiarize dentists with the positive role of the PT in CMD therapy. The three main chapters each start with a textual description, then provide extensive black and white clinical photographs illustrating the concepts covered. Topics include protocol; treatment of hypermobility, hypomobility, **bruxism,** and the abused protrusion; and specific problems, including the anterior displacement of the temporomandibular joint (TMJ) disc without reduction, postoperative pain, osteoarthritis, and acute TMJ arthritis. The authors focus on the pure mechanical corrections for determined unilateral overloading of the stomatognathic system. The authors emphasize that the patient should be actively involved in the treatment with the emphasis at first on posture, stretching, and strengthening. One appendix provides recordkeeping forms for the physical therapy examination. 144 figures. 18 references. (AA-M).

- **Prevention and Treatment Considerations for the Dental Patient With Special Needs**

Source: Academy of Dentistry for Persons with Disabilities, American Academy of Pediatric Dentistry. 199x. 89 p.

Contact: Available from American Dental Hygienists' Association (ADHA). 444 North Michigan Avenue, Chicago, IL 60611. (800) 243-2342 or (312) 440-8900; Fax (312) 440-8929; E-mail: adha@ix.netcom.com; http://www.adha.org. PRICE: $2.00 for booklet, $15.00 for slides (30-day rental only, plus $50.00 refundable deposit); nonmembers add 25 percent (Illinois residents add 8 percent sales tax). Order number 2933.

Summary: This manual includes a basic discussion of prevention and treatment considerations for dental patients with special needs. Topics covered include quality of life; dietary considerations; plaque; periodontal disease; nursing-related caries (baby bottle tooth decay); the sugar content of medications; phenytoin (Dilantin); over-retained teeth; **bruxism;** drooling; mastication, rumination, and pouching; mental retardation; the Down Syndrome pattern of tooth eruption; dental implications of cerebral palsy; orthodontic therapy; trauma; self-injurious behavior; physical and sexual abuse; restraint and management; supporting devices; toothbrushing, including positioning techniques; preventive agents; adaptive equipment; and psychosocial factors. The manual concludes with a glossary of terms for the use of non-dental professionals, a list of resources, and a bibliography. Black and white photographs illustrate many of the conditions discussed. 45 references.

Chapters on Bruxism

In order to find chapters that specifically relate to bruxism, an excellent source of abstracts is the Combined Health Information Database. You will need to limit your search to book chapters and bruxism using the "Detailed Search" option. Go to the following hyperlink: **http://chid.nih.gov/detail/detail.html**. To find book chapters, use the drop boxes at the bottom of the search page where "You may refine your search by." Select the dates and language you prefer, and the format option "Book Chapter." Type "bruxism" (or synonyms) into the "For these words:" box. The following is a typical result when searching for book chapters on bruxism:

- **Bruxism**

  Source: in Sutton, A.L. Dental Care and Oral Health Sourcebook. 2nd ed. Detroit, MI: Omnigraphics. 2003. p. 369-372.

  Contact: Available from Omnigraphics. 615 Griswold Street, Detroit, MI 48226. (313) 961-1340. Fax: (313) 961-1383. E-mail: progers@omnigraphics.com. www.omnigraphics.com. PRICE: $78.00; plus shipping and handling. ISBN: 780806344.

  Summary: Bruxism is the medical term for the grinding of teeth or the clenching of jaws, especially during deep sleep or while under stress. This chapter on **bruxism** is from a book that provides information about dental care and oral health at all stages of life. Topics include a definition of **bruxism**, the causes of **bruxism**, complications or problems associated with the condition, diagnostic considerations, prevention strategies, and treatment options, including relaxation methods. The author focuses on **bruxism** in children.

CHAPTER 5. MULTIMEDIA ON BRUXISM

Overview

In this chapter, we show you how to keep current on multimedia sources of information on bruxism. We start with sources that have been summarized by federal agencies, and then show you how to find bibliographic information catalogued by the National Library of Medicine.

Video Recordings

An excellent source of multimedia information on bruxism is the Combined Health Information Database. You will need to limit your search to "Videorecording" and "bruxism" using the "Detailed Search" option. Go directly to the following hyperlink: **http://chid.nih.gov/detail/detail.html**. To find video productions, use the drop boxes at the bottom of the search page where "You may refine your search by." Select the dates and language you prefer, and the format option "Videorecording (videotape, videocassette, etc.)." Type "bruxism" (or synonyms) into the "For these words:" box. The following is a typical result when searching for video recordings on bruxism:

- **Oral Care Management of Persons with Movement Disorders**

    Source: Seattle, WA: Dental Education in Care of Persons with Disabilities (DECOD), University of Washington. 1997. (videocassette).

    Contact: Available from Dental Education in Care of Persons with Disabilities (DECOD). Continuing Dental Education, Box 357137, University of Washington, Seattle, WA 98195-6370. (206) 543-5448. Fax (206) 685-3164. PRICE: $95.00 plus shipping and handling.

    Summary: For persons with movement disorders, maintaining oral health can make a significant difference in their quality of life. Yet, the provision of oral health care to persons with such conditions can be a challenge for the patient, the caregiver, and the dental professional. This videotape is designed for audiences who wish to learn more about oral home care as well as for those treating patients with unanticipated or uncontrolled movements in the dental office setting. Filmed in dental clinic settings with actual patients, the program covers oral care for persons with an array of neuromotor dysfunctions, including cerebral palsy, multiple sclerosis, amyotrophic lateral sclerosis, spinal cord injury, Parkinson's disease, and chronic mental illness. The program addresses issues in communication, positioning, control of pain and anxiety, primitive reflexes, airway protection, stabilization of the head, **bruxism,** oral hygiene, and use of oral chemotherapeutic agents and adaptive aides. In each of these areas, effective management techniques are demonstrated. The program also offers practical instruction in methods of preventive oral care for persons with self-care ability as well as those dependent on caregivers. (AA-M).

- **Dental Care for Individuals with Cerebral Palsy**

  Source: Indianapolis, IN: United Cerebral Palsy Association of Greater Indiana, Inc. 199x. (videocassette).

  Contact: Available from United Cerebral Palsy Association of Greater Indiana, Inc. 615 North Alabama Street, Room 322, Indianapolis, IN 46204. (317) 632-3561. PRICE: $30.00 each; free for Indiana residents.

  Summary: This videotape program provides parents with information about dental care and oral hygiene for children with cerebral palsy (CP). Narrated by Dr. Brian Sanders, DDS, the program reviews the dental conditions associated with CP and explains how parents can improve the quality of home and dental care provided to children with CP. The program stresses that it can be difficult to find time for proper dental care, that children with CP can be 'orally defensive', and that some of the related medical care (drugs and special diets) can be risk factors for increased oral health problems in these children. The program then reviews common questions that parents may have, providing basic answers to those questions. Topics include finding a dentist who will treat the child with CP, the child's first visit to the dentist, bottle-feeding concerns, managing special diets (especially those that are high in sugars), caries rate and gingival (gum) problems, preparing the child for a dental visit, handling dental visits that do not go well, toothbrushing techniques (including managing the increased gag reflex in these children), the use of mouth props and or restraints for dental care, braces, toothgrinding (bruxism), mouthguards, seizures, and falls or trauma to the mouth and face. The video depicts children with CP at the dental office and at home, experiencing toothbrushing or dental examinations.

CHAPTER 6. PERIODICALS AND NEWS ON BRUXISM

Overview

In this chapter, we suggest a number of news sources and present various periodicals that cover bruxism.

News Services and Press Releases

One of the simplest ways of tracking press releases on bruxism is to search the news wires. In the following sample of sources, we will briefly describe how to access each service. These services only post recent news intended for public viewing.

PR Newswire

To access the PR Newswire archive, simply go to **http://www.prnewswire.com/**. Select your country. Type "bruxism" (or synonyms) into the search box. You will automatically receive information on relevant news releases posted within the last 30 days. The search results are shown by order of relevance.

Reuters Health

The Reuters' Medical News and Health eLine databases can be very useful in exploring news archives relating to bruxism. While some of the listed articles are free to view, others are available for purchase for a nominal fee. To access this archive, go to **http://www.reutershealth.com/en/index.html** and search by "bruxism" (or synonyms). The following was recently listed in this archive for bruxism:

- **Sleep bruxism associated with obstructive sleep apnea**
  Source: Reuters Medical News
  Date: January 23, 2001

The NIH

Within MEDLINEplus, the NIH has made an agreement with the New York Times Syndicate, the AP News Service, and Reuters to deliver news that can be browsed by the public. Search news releases at **http://www.nlm.nih.gov/medlineplus/alphanews_a.html**. MEDLINEplus allows you to browse across an alphabetical index. Or you can search by date at the following Web page: **http://www.nlm.nih.gov/medlineplus/newsbydate.html**. Often, news items are indexed by MEDLINEplus within its search engine.

Business Wire

Business Wire is similar to PR Newswire. To access this archive, simply go to **http://www.businesswire.com/**. You can scan the news by industry category or company name.

Market Wire

Market Wire is more focused on technology than the other wires. To browse the latest press releases by topic, such as alternative medicine, biotechnology, fitness, healthcare, legal, nutrition, and pharmaceuticals, access Market Wire's Medical/Health channel at **http://www.marketwire.com/mw/release_index?channel=MedicalHealth**. Or simply go to Market Wire's home page at **http://www.marketwire.com/mw/home**, type "bruxism" (or synonyms) into the search box, and click on "Search News." As this service is technology oriented, you may wish to use it when searching for press releases covering diagnostic procedures or tests.

Search Engines

Medical news is also available in the news sections of commercial Internet search engines. See the health news page at Yahoo (**http://dir.yahoo.com/Health/News_and_Media/**), or you can use this Web site's general news search page at **http://news.yahoo.com/**. Type in "bruxism" (or synonyms). If you know the name of a company that is relevant to bruxism, you can go to any stock trading Web site (such as **http://www.etrade.com/**) and search for the company name there. News items across various news sources are reported on indicated hyperlinks. Google offers a similar service at **http://news.google.com/**.

BBC

Covering news from a more European perspective, the British Broadcasting Corporation (BBC) allows the public free access to their news archive located at **http://www.bbc.co.uk/**. Search by "bruxism" (or synonyms).

Newsletter Articles

Use the Combined Health Information Database, and limit your search criteria to "newsletter articles." Again, you will need to use the "Detailed Search" option. Go directly to the following hyperlink: **http://chid.nih.gov/detail/detail.html**. Go to the bottom of the search page where "You may refine your search by." Select the dates and language that you prefer. For the format option, select "Newsletter Article." Type "bruxism" (or synonyms) into the "For these words:" box. You should check back periodically with this database as it is updated every three months. The following is a typical result when searching for newsletter articles on bruxism:

- **Jaw Problems**

    Source: Mayo Clinic Health Letter. 20(6): 6. January 2002.

    Contact: Available from Mayo Clinic Health Letter. 200 First Street SW, Rochester, MN 55905. (800) 333-9037 or (303) 604-1465. Email: HealthLetter@Mayo.Edu.

    Summary: This newsletter article for patients describes symptoms and treatment of temporomandibular disorders. The temporomandibular joints (TMJ) are the joints that connect the lower jawbones to the temporal bone of the skull. Acute and chronic pain occurs when these joints or the muscles surrounding these joints are injured. Tenderness, aching, clicking sounds or grating sensations, locking of the jaw, and headaches or earaches are symptoms of temporomandibular disorders. These symptoms can be caused by osteoarthritis of the jaw, major injury to the jaw, and minor trauma caused by **bruxism,** chewing gum, or clenching the teeth. Treatments for this disorder include NSAIDS, dental aids, physical therapy, and patient education techniques that include avoiding habits that cause pain to the jaw, regular exercise, and adequate sleep. Surgery may be needed if other treatments are unsuccessful.

Academic Periodicals covering Bruxism

Numerous periodicals are currently indexed within the National Library of Medicine's PubMed database that are known to publish articles relating to bruxism. In addition to these sources, you can search for articles covering bruxism that have been published by any of the periodicals listed in previous chapters. To find the latest studies published, go to **http://www.ncbi.nlm.nih.gov/pubmed**, type the name of the periodical into the search box, and click "Go."

If you want complete details about the historical contents of a journal, you can also visit the following Web site: **http://www.ncbi.nlm.nih.gov/entrez/jrbrowser.cgi**. Here, type in the name of the journal or its abbreviation, and you will receive an index of published articles. At **http://locatorplus.gov/**, you can retrieve more indexing information on medical periodicals (e.g. the name of the publisher). Select the button "Search LOCATORplus." Then type in the name of the journal and select the advanced search option "Journal Title Search."

APPENDICES

APPENDIX A. PHYSICIAN RESOURCES

Overview

In this chapter, we focus on databases and Internet-based guidelines and information resources created or written for a professional audience.

NIH Guidelines

Commonly referred to as "clinical" or "professional" guidelines, the National Institutes of Health publish physician guidelines for the most common diseases. Publications are available at the following by relevant Institute[6]:

- Office of the Director (OD); guidelines consolidated across agencies available at **http://www.nih.gov/health/consumer/conkey.htm**

- National Institute of General Medical Sciences (NIGMS); fact sheets available at **http://www.nigms.nih.gov/news/facts/**

- National Library of Medicine (NLM); extensive encyclopedia (A.D.A.M., Inc.) with guidelines: **http://www.nlm.nih.gov/medlineplus/healthtopics.html**

- National Cancer Institute (NCI); guidelines available at **http://www.cancer.gov/cancerinfo/list.aspx?viewid=5f35036e-5497-4d86-8c2c-714a9f7c8d25**

- National Eye Institute (NEI); guidelines available at **http://www.nei.nih.gov/order/index.htm**

- National Heart, Lung, and Blood Institute (NHLBI); guidelines available at **http://www.nhlbi.nih.gov/guidelines/index.htm**

- National Human Genome Research Institute (NHGRI); research available at **http://www.genome.gov/page.cfm?pageID=10000375**

- National Institute on Aging (NIA); guidelines available at **http://www.nia.nih.gov/health/**

---

[6] These publications are typically written by one or more of the various NIH Institutes.

- National Institute on Alcohol Abuse and Alcoholism (NIAAA); guidelines available at http://www.niaaa.nih.gov/publications/publications.htm

- National Institute of Allergy and Infectious Diseases (NIAID); guidelines available at http://www.niaid.nih.gov/publications/

- National Institute of Arthritis and Musculoskeletal and Skin Diseases (NIAMS); fact sheets and guidelines available at http://www.niams.nih.gov/hi/index.htm

- National Institute of Child Health and Human Development (NICHD); guidelines available at http://www.nichd.nih.gov/publications/pubskey.cfm

- National Institute on Deafness and Other Communication Disorders (NIDCD); fact sheets and guidelines at http://www.nidcd.nih.gov/health/

- National Institute of Dental and Craniofacial Research (NIDCR); guidelines available at http://www.nidr.nih.gov/health/

- National Institute of Diabetes and Digestive and Kidney Diseases (NIDDK); guidelines available at http://www.niddk.nih.gov/health/health.htm

- National Institute on Drug Abuse (NIDA); guidelines available at http://www.nida.nih.gov/DrugAbuse.html

- National Institute of Environmental Health Sciences (NIEHS); environmental health information available at http://www.niehs.nih.gov/external/facts.htm

- National Institute of Mental Health (NIMH); guidelines available at http://www.nimh.nih.gov/practitioners/index.cfm

- National Institute of Neurological Disorders and Stroke (NINDS); neurological disorder information pages available at http://www.ninds.nih.gov/health_and_medical/disorder_index.htm

- National Institute of Nursing Research (NINR); publications on selected illnesses at http://www.nih.gov/ninr/news-info/publications.html

- National Institute of Biomedical Imaging and Bioengineering; general information at http://grants.nih.gov/grants/becon/becon_info.htm

- Center for Information Technology (CIT); referrals to other agencies based on keyword searches available at http://kb.nih.gov/www_query_main.asp

- National Center for Complementary and Alternative Medicine (NCCAM); health information available at http://nccam.nih.gov/health/

- National Center for Research Resources (NCRR); various information directories available at http://www.ncrr.nih.gov/publications.asp

- Office of Rare Diseases; various fact sheets available at http://rarediseases.info.nih.gov/html/resources/rep_pubs.html

- Centers for Disease Control and Prevention; various fact sheets on infectious diseases available at http://www.cdc.gov/publications.htm

NIH Databases

In addition to the various Institutes of Health that publish professional guidelines, the NIH has designed a number of databases for professionals.[7] Physician-oriented resources provide a wide variety of information related to the biomedical and health sciences, both past and present. The format of these resources varies. Searchable databases, bibliographic citations, full-text articles (when available), archival collections, and images are all available. The following are referenced by the National Library of Medicine:[8]

- **Bioethics:** Access to published literature on the ethical, legal, and public policy issues surrounding healthcare and biomedical research. This information is provided in conjunction with the Kennedy Institute of Ethics located at Georgetown University, Washington, D.C.: **http://www.nlm.nih.gov/databases/databases_bioethics.html**

- **HIV/AIDS Resources:** Describes various links and databases dedicated to HIV/AIDS research: **http://www.nlm.nih.gov/pubs/factsheets/aidsinfs.html**

- **NLM Online Exhibitions:** Describes "Exhibitions in the History of Medicine": **http://www.nlm.nih.gov/exhibition/exhibition.html**. Additional resources for historical scholarship in medicine: **http://www.nlm.nih.gov/hmd/hmd.html**

- **Biotechnology Information:** Access to public databases. The National Center for Biotechnology Information conducts research in computational biology, develops software tools for analyzing genome data, and disseminates biomedical information for the better understanding of molecular processes affecting human health and disease: **http://www.ncbi.nlm.nih.gov/**

- **Population Information:** The National Library of Medicine provides access to worldwide coverage of population, family planning, and related health issues, including family planning technology and programs, fertility, and population law and policy: **http://www.nlm.nih.gov/databases/databases_population.html**

- **Cancer Information:** Access to cancer-oriented databases: **http://www.nlm.nih.gov/databases/databases_cancer.html**

- **Profiles in Science:** Offering the archival collections of prominent twentieth-century biomedical scientists to the public through modern digital technology: **http://www.profiles.nlm.nih.gov/**

- **Chemical Information:** Provides links to various chemical databases and references: **http://sis.nlm.nih.gov/Chem/ChemMain.html**

- **Clinical Alerts:** Reports the release of findings from the NIH-funded clinical trials where such release could significantly affect morbidity and mortality: **http://www.nlm.nih.gov/databases/alerts/clinical_alerts.html**

- **Space Life Sciences:** Provides links and information to space-based research (including NASA): **http://www.nlm.nih.gov/databases/databases_space.html**

- **MEDLINE:** Bibliographic database covering the fields of medicine, nursing, dentistry, veterinary medicine, the healthcare system, and the pre-clinical sciences: **http://www.nlm.nih.gov/databases/databases_medline.html**

---

[7] Remember, for the general public, the National Library of Medicine recommends the databases referenced in MEDLINE*plus* (**http://medlineplus.gov/** or **http://www.nlm.nih.gov/medlineplus/databases.html**).

[8] See **http://www.nlm.nih.gov/databases/databases.html**.

- **Toxicology and Environmental Health Information (TOXNET):** Databases covering toxicology and environmental health: **http://sis.nlm.nih.gov/Tox/ToxMain.html**

- **Visible Human Interface:** Anatomically detailed, three-dimensional representations of normal male and female human bodies: **http://www.nlm.nih.gov/research/visible/visible_human.html**

The NLM Gateway[9]

The NLM (National Library of Medicine) Gateway is a Web-based system that lets users search simultaneously in multiple retrieval systems at the U.S. National Library of Medicine (NLM). It allows users of NLM services to initiate searches from one Web interface, providing one-stop searching for many of NLM's information resources or databases.[10] To use the NLM Gateway, simply go to the search site at **http://gateway.nlm.nih.gov/gw/Cmd**. Type "bruxism" (or synonyms) into the search box and click "Search." The results will be presented in a tabular form, indicating the number of references in each database category.

Results Summary

Category	Items Found
Journal Articles	1737
Books / Periodicals / Audio Visual	12
Consumer Health	1
Meeting Abstracts	1
Other Collections	26
Total	1777

HSTAT[11]

HSTAT is a free, Web-based resource that provides access to full-text documents used in healthcare decision-making.[12] These documents include clinical practice guidelines, quick-reference guides for clinicians, consumer health brochures, evidence reports and technology assessments from the Agency for Healthcare Research and Quality (AHRQ), as well as AHRQ's Put Prevention Into Practice.[13] Simply search by "bruxism" (or synonyms) at the following Web site: **http://text.nlm.nih.gov**.

---

[9] Adapted from NLM: **http://gateway.nlm.nih.gov/gw/Cmd?Overview.x**.

[10] The NLM Gateway is currently being developed by the Lister Hill National Center for Biomedical Communications (LHNCBC) at the National Library of Medicine (NLM) of the National Institutes of Health (NIH).

[11] Adapted from HSTAT: **http://www.nlm.nih.gov/pubs/factsheets/hstat.html**.

[12] The HSTAT URL is **http://hstat.nlm.nih.gov/**.

[13] Other important documents in HSTAT include: the National Institutes of Health (NIH) Consensus Conference Reports and Technology Assessment Reports; the HIV/AIDS Treatment Information Service (ATIS) resource documents; the Substance Abuse and Mental Health Services Administration's Center for Substance Abuse Treatment (SAMHSA/CSAT) Treatment Improvement Protocols (TIP) and Center for Substance Abuse Prevention (SAMHSA/CSAP) Prevention Enhancement Protocols System (PEPS); the Public Health Service (PHS) Preventive Services Task Force's *Guide to Clinical Preventive Services*; the independent, nonfederal Task Force on Community Services' *Guide to Community Preventive Services*; and the Health Technology Advisory Committee (HTAC) of the Minnesota Health Care Commission (MHCC) health technology evaluations.

Coffee Break: Tutorials for Biologists[14]

Coffee Break is a general healthcare site that takes a scientific view of the news and covers recent breakthroughs in biology that may one day assist physicians in developing treatments. Here you will find a collection of short reports on recent biological discoveries. Each report incorporates interactive tutorials that demonstrate how bioinformatics tools are used as a part of the research process. Currently, all Coffee Breaks are written by NCBI staff.[15] Each report is about 400 words and is usually based on a discovery reported in one or more articles from recently published, peer-reviewed literature.[16] This site has new articles every few weeks, so it can be considered an online magazine of sorts. It is intended for general background information. You can access the Coffee Break Web site at the following hyperlink: **http://www.ncbi.nlm.nih.gov/Coffeebreak/**.

Other Commercial Databases

In addition to resources maintained by official agencies, other databases exist that are commercial ventures addressing medical professionals. Here are some examples that may interest you:

- **CliniWeb International:** Index and table of contents to selected clinical information on the Internet; see **http://www.ohsu.edu/cliniweb/**.

- **Medical World Search:** Searches full text from thousands of selected medical sites on the Internet; see **http://www.mwsearch.com/**.

---

[14] Adapted from **http://www.ncbi.nlm.nih.gov/Coffeebreak/Archive/FAQ.html**.

[15] The figure that accompanies each article is frequently supplied by an expert external to NCBI, in which case the source of the figure is cited. The result is an interactive tutorial that tells a biological story.

[16] After a brief introduction that sets the work described into a broader context, the report focuses on how a molecular understanding can provide explanations of observed biology and lead to therapies for diseases. Each vignette is accompanied by a figure and hypertext links that lead to a series of pages that interactively show how NCBI tools and resources are used in the research process.

APPENDIX B. PATIENT RESOURCES

Overview

Official agencies, as well as federally funded institutions supported by national grants, frequently publish a variety of guidelines written with the patient in mind. These are typically called "Fact Sheets" or "Guidelines." They can take the form of a brochure, information kit, pamphlet, or flyer. Often they are only a few pages in length. Since new guidelines on bruxism can appear at any moment and be published by a number of sources, the best approach to finding guidelines is to systematically scan the Internet-based services that post them.

Patient Guideline Sources

The remainder of this chapter directs you to sources which either publish or can help you find additional guidelines on topics related to bruxism. Due to space limitations, these sources are listed in a concise manner. Do not hesitate to consult the following sources by either using the Internet hyperlink provided, or, in cases where the contact information is provided, contacting the publisher or author directly.

The National Institutes of Health

The NIH gateway to patients is located at **http://health.nih.gov/**. From this site, you can search across various sources and institutes, a number of which are summarized below.

Topic Pages: MEDLINEplus

The National Library of Medicine has created a vast and patient-oriented healthcare information portal called MEDLINEplus. Within this Internet-based system are "health topic pages" which list links to available materials relevant to bruxism. To access this system, log on to **http://www.nlm.nih.gov/medlineplus/healthtopics.html**. From there you can either search using the alphabetical index or browse by broad topic areas. Recently, MEDLINEplus listed the following when searched for "bruxism":

Anatomy
http://www.nlm.nih.gov/medlineplus/anatomy.html

Child Dental Health
http://www.nlm.nih.gov/medlineplus/childdentalhealth.html

Cosmetic Dentistry
http://www.nlm.nih.gov/medlineplus/cosmeticdentistry.html

Dental Health
http://www.nlm.nih.gov/medlineplus/dentalhealth.html

Gum Disease
http://www.nlm.nih.gov/medlineplus/gumdisease.html

Orthodontia
http://www.nlm.nih.gov/medlineplus/orthodontia.html

Sleep Disorders
http://www.nlm.nih.gov/medlineplus/sleepdisorders.html

Temporomandibular Joint Dysfunction
http://www.nlm.nih.gov/medlineplus/temporomandibularjointdysfunction.html

Tooth Disorders
http://www.nlm.nih.gov/medlineplus/toothdisorders.html

You may also choose to use the search utility provided by MEDLINEplus at the following Web address: **http://www.nlm.nih.gov/medlineplus/**. Simply type a keyword into the search box and click "Search." This utility is similar to the NIH search utility, with the exception that it only includes materials that are linked within the MEDLINEplus system (mostly patient-oriented information). It also has the disadvantage of generating unstructured results. We recommend, therefore, that you use this method only if you have a very targeted search.

The Combined Health Information Database (CHID)

CHID Online is a reference tool that maintains a database directory of thousands of journal articles and patient education guidelines on bruxism. CHID offers summaries that describe the guidelines available, including contact information and pricing. CHID's general Web site is **http://chid.nih.gov/**. To search this database, go to **http://chid.nih.gov/detail/detail.html**. In particular, you can use the advanced search options to look up pamphlets, reports, brochures, and information kits. The following was recently posted in this archive:

- **Tooth Grinding (Bruxism)**

  Source: in Griffith, H.W. Instruction for Patients. 5th ed. Orlando, FL: W.B. Saunders Company. 1994. p. 471.

  Contact: Available from W.B. Saunders Company. Order Fulfillment, 6277 Sea Harbor Drive, Orlando, FL 32887-4430. (800) 545-2522 (individuals) or (800) 782-4479 (schools); Fax (800) 874-6418 or (407) 352-3445; http://www.wbsaunders.com. PRICE: $52.00 (English); $49.95 (Spanish); plus shipping and handling. ISBN: 0721649300 (English); 0721669972 (Spanish).

Summary: This fact sheet on **bruxism** (toothgrinding) is from a compilation of instructions for patients, published in book format. The fact sheet provides information in three sections: basic information, including a description of the condition, frequent signs and symptoms, causes, risk factors, preventive measures, expected outcome, and possible complications; treatment, including general measures, medication, activity guidelines, and diet; and when to contact one's health care provider. The fact sheet is designed to be photocopied and distributed to patients as a reinforcement of oral instructions and as a teaching tool.

The NIH Search Utility

The NIH search utility allows you to search for documents on over 100 selected Web sites that comprise the NIH-WEB-SPACE. Each of these servers is "crawled" and indexed on an ongoing basis. Your search will produce a list of various documents, all of which will relate in some way to bruxism. The drawbacks of this approach are that the information is not organized by theme and that the references are often a mix of information for professionals and patients. Nevertheless, a large number of the listed Web sites provide useful background information. We can only recommend this route, therefore, for relatively rare or specific disorders, or when using highly targeted searches. To use the NIH search utility, visit the following Web page: **http://search.nih.gov/index.html**.

Additional Web Sources

A number of Web sites are available to the public that often link to government sites. These can also point you in the direction of essential information. The following is a representative sample:

- AOL: **http://search.aol.com/cat.adp?id=168&layer=&from=subcats**

- Family Village: **http://www.familyvillage.wisc.edu/specific.htm**

- Google: **http://directory.google.com/Top/Health/Conditions_and_Diseases/**

- Med Help International: **http://www.medhelp.org/HealthTopics/A.html**

- Open Directory Project: **http://dmoz.org/Health/Conditions_and_Diseases/**

- Yahoo.com: **http://dir.yahoo.com/Health/Diseases_and_Conditions/**

- WebMD®Health: **http://my.webmd.com/health_topics**

Finding Associations

There are several Internet directories that provide lists of medical associations with information on or resources relating to bruxism. By consulting all of associations listed in this chapter, you will have nearly exhausted all sources for patient associations concerned with bruxism.

The National Health Information Center (NHIC)

The National Health Information Center (NHIC) offers a free referral service to help people find organizations that provide information about bruxism. For more information, see the

NHIC's Web site at **http://www.health.gov/NHIC/** or contact an information specialist by calling 1-800-336-4797.

Directory of Health Organizations

The Directory of Health Organizations, provided by the National Library of Medicine Specialized Information Services, is a comprehensive source of information on associations. The Directory of Health Organizations database can be accessed via the Internet at **http://www.sis.nlm.nih.gov/Dir/DirMain.html**. It is composed of two parts: DIRLINE and Health Hotlines.

The DIRLINE database comprises some 10,000 records of organizations, research centers, and government institutes and associations that primarily focus on health and biomedicine. To access DIRLINE directly, go to the following Web site: **http://dirline.nlm.nih.gov/**. Simply type in "bruxism" (or a synonym), and you will receive information on all relevant organizations listed in the database.

Health Hotlines directs you to toll-free numbers to over 300 organizations. You can access this database directly at **http://www.sis.nlm.nih.gov/hotlines/**. On this page, you are given the option to search by keyword or by browsing the subject list. When you have received your search results, click on the name of the organization for its description and contact information.

The Combined Health Information Database

Another comprehensive source of information on healthcare associations is the Combined Health Information Database. Using the "Detailed Search" option, you will need to limit your search to "Organizations" and "bruxism". Type the following hyperlink into your Web browser: **http://chid.nih.gov/detail/detail.html**. To find associations, use the drop boxes at the bottom of the search page where "You may refine your search by." For publication date, select "All Years." Then, select your preferred language and the format option "Organization Resource Sheet." Type "bruxism" (or synonyms) into the "For these words:" box. You should check back periodically with this database since it is updated every three months.

The National Organization for Rare Disorders, Inc.

The National Organization for Rare Disorders, Inc. has prepared a Web site that provides, at no charge, lists of associations organized by health topic. You can access this database at the following Web site: **http://www.rarediseases.org/search/orgsearch.html**. Type "bruxism" (or a synonym) into the search box, and click "Submit Query."

APPENDIX C. FINDING MEDICAL LIBRARIES

Overview

In this Appendix, we show you how to quickly find a medical library in your area.

Preparation

Your local public library and medical libraries have interlibrary loan programs with the National Library of Medicine (NLM), one of the largest medical collections in the world. According to the NLM, most of the literature in the general and historical collections of the National Library of Medicine is available on interlibrary loan to any library. If you would like to access NLM medical literature, then visit a library in your area that can request the publications for you.[17]

Finding a Local Medical Library

The quickest method to locate medical libraries is to use the Internet-based directory published by the National Network of Libraries of Medicine (NN/LM). This network includes 4626 members and affiliates that provide many services to librarians, health professionals, and the public. To find a library in your area, simply visit **http://nnlm.gov/members/adv.html** or call 1-800-338-7657.

Medical Libraries in the U.S. and Canada

In addition to the NN/LM, the National Library of Medicine (NLM) lists a number of libraries with reference facilities that are open to the public. The following is the NLM's list and includes hyperlinks to each library's Web site. These Web pages can provide information on hours of operation and other restrictions. The list below is a small sample of

---

[17] Adapted from the NLM: **http://www.nlm.nih.gov/psd/cas/interlibrary.html**.

libraries recommended by the National Library of Medicine (sorted alphabetically by name of the U.S. state or Canadian province where the library is located)[18]:

- **Alabama:** Health InfoNet of Jefferson County (Jefferson County Library Cooperative, Lister Hill Library of the Health Sciences), **http://www.uab.edu/infonet/**

- **Alabama:** Richard M. Scrushy Library (American Sports Medicine Institute)

- **Arizona:** Samaritan Regional Medical Center: The Learning Center (Samaritan Health System, Phoenix, Arizona), **http://www.samaritan.edu/library/bannerlibs.htm**

- **California:** Kris Kelly Health Information Center (St. Joseph Health System, Humboldt), **http://www.humboldt1.com/~kkhic/index.html**

- **California:** Community Health Library of Los Gatos, **http://www.healthlib.org/orgresources.html**

- **California:** Consumer Health Program and Services (CHIPS) (County of Los Angeles Public Library, Los Angeles County Harbor-UCLA Medical Center Library) - Carson, CA, **http://www.colapublib.org/services/chips.html**

- **California:** Gateway Health Library (Sutter Gould Medical Foundation)

- **California:** Health Library (Stanford University Medical Center), **http://www-med.stanford.edu/healthlibrary/**

- **California:** Patient Education Resource Center - Health Information and Resources (University of California, San Francisco), **http://sfghdean.ucsf.edu/barnett/PERC/default.asp**

- **California:** Redwood Health Library (Petaluma Health Care District), **http://www.phcd.org/rdwdlib.html**

- **California:** Los Gatos PlaneTree Health Library, **http://planetreesanjose.org/**

- **California:** Sutter Resource Library (Sutter Hospitals Foundation, Sacramento), **http://suttermedicalcenter.org/library/**

- **California:** Health Sciences Libraries (University of California, Davis), **http://www.lib.ucdavis.edu/healthsci/**

- **California:** ValleyCare Health Library & Ryan Comer Cancer Resource Center (ValleyCare Health System, Pleasanton), **http://gaelnet.stmarys-ca.edu/other.libs/gbal/east/vchl.html**

- **California:** Washington Community Health Resource Library (Fremont), **http://www.healthlibrary.org/**

- **Colorado:** William V. Gervasini Memorial Library (Exempla Healthcare), **http://www.saintjosephdenver.org/yourhealth/libraries/**

- **Connecticut:** Hartford Hospital Health Science Libraries (Hartford Hospital), **http://www.harthosp.org/library/**

- **Connecticut:** Healthnet: Connecticut Consumer Health Information Center (University of Connecticut Health Center, Lyman Maynard Stowe Library), **http://library.uchc.edu/departm/hnet/**

---

[18] Abstracted from **http://www.nlm.nih.gov/medlineplus/libraries.html**.

- **Connecticut:** Waterbury Hospital Health Center Library (Waterbury Hospital, Waterbury), **http://www.waterburyhospital.com/library/consumer.shtml**

- **Delaware:** Consumer Health Library (Christiana Care Health System, Eugene du Pont Preventive Medicine & Rehabilitation Institute, Wilmington), **http://www.christianacare.org/health_guide/health_guide_pmri_health_info.cfm**

- **Delaware:** Lewis B. Flinn Library (Delaware Academy of Medicine, Wilmington), **http://www.delamed.org/chls.html**

- **Georgia:** Family Resource Library (Medical College of Georgia, Augusta), **http://cmc.mcg.edu/kids_families/fam_resources/fam_res_lib/frl.htm**

- **Georgia:** Health Resource Center (Medical Center of Central Georgia, Macon), **http://www.mccg.org/hrc/hrchome.asp**

- **Hawaii:** Hawaii Medical Library: Consumer Health Information Service (Hawaii Medical Library, Honolulu), **http://hml.org/CHIS/**

- **Idaho:** DeArmond Consumer Health Library (Kootenai Medical Center, Coeur d'Alene), **http://www.nicon.org/DeArmond/index.htm**

- **Illinois:** Health Learning Center of Northwestern Memorial Hospital (Chicago), **http://www.nmh.org/health_info/hlc.html**

- **Illinois:** Medical Library (OSF Saint Francis Medical Center, Peoria), **http://www.osfsaintfrancis.org/general/library/**

- **Kentucky:** Medical Library - Services for Patients, Families, Students & the Public (Central Baptist Hospital, Lexington), **http://www.centralbap.com/education/community/library.cfm**

- **Kentucky:** University of Kentucky - Health Information Library (Chandler Medical Center, Lexington), **http://www.mc.uky.edu/PatientEd/**

- **Louisiana:** Alton Ochsner Medical Foundation Library (Alton Ochsner Medical Foundation, New Orleans), **http://www.ochsner.org/library/**

- **Louisiana:** Louisiana State University Health Sciences Center Medical Library-Shreveport, **http://lib-sh.lsuhsc.edu/**

- **Maine:** Franklin Memorial Hospital Medical Library (Franklin Memorial Hospital, Farmington), **http://www.fchn.org/fmh/lib.htm**

- **Maine:** Gerrish-True Health Sciences Library (Central Maine Medical Center, Lewiston), **http://www.cmmc.org/library/library.html**

- **Maine:** Hadley Parrot Health Science Library (Eastern Maine Healthcare, Bangor), **http://www.emh.org/hll/hpl/guide.htm**

- **Maine:** Maine Medical Center Library (Maine Medical Center, Portland), **http://www.mmc.org/library/**

- **Maine:** Parkview Hospital (Brunswick), **http://www.parkviewhospital.org/**

- **Maine:** Southern Maine Medical Center Health Sciences Library (Southern Maine Medical Center, Biddeford), **http://www.smmc.org/services/service.php3?choice=10**

- **Maine:** Stephens Memorial Hospital's Health Information Library (Western Maine Health, Norway), **http://www.wmhcc.org/Library/**

- **Manitoba, Canada:** Consumer & Patient Health Information Service (University of Manitoba Libraries), http://www.umanitoba.ca/libraries/units/health/reference/chis.html

- **Manitoba, Canada:** J.W. Crane Memorial Library (Deer Lodge Centre, Winnipeg), http://www.deerlodge.mb.ca/crane_library/about.asp

- **Maryland:** Health Information Center at the Wheaton Regional Library (Montgomery County, Dept. of Public Libraries, Wheaton Regional Library), http://www.mont.lib.md.us/healthinfo/hic.asp

- **Massachusetts:** Baystate Medical Center Library (Baystate Health System), http://www.baystatehealth.com/1024/

- **Massachusetts:** Boston University Medical Center Alumni Medical Library (Boston University Medical Center), http://med-libwww.bu.edu/library/lib.html

- **Massachusetts:** Lowell General Hospital Health Sciences Library (Lowell General Hospital, Lowell), http://www.lowellgeneral.org/library/HomePageLinks/WWW.htm

- **Massachusetts:** Paul E. Woodard Health Sciences Library (New England Baptist Hospital, Boston), http://www.nebh.org/health_lib.asp

- **Massachusetts:** St. Luke's Hospital Health Sciences Library (St. Luke's Hospital, Southcoast Health System, New Bedford), http://www.southcoast.org/library/

- **Massachusetts:** Treadwell Library Consumer Health Reference Center (Massachusetts General Hospital), http://www.mgh.harvard.edu/library/chrcindex.html

- **Massachusetts:** UMass HealthNet (University of Massachusetts Medical School, Worchester), http://healthnet.umassmed.edu/

- **Michigan:** Botsford General Hospital Library - Consumer Health (Botsford General Hospital, Library & Internet Services), http://www.botsfordlibrary.org/consumer.htm

- **Michigan:** Helen DeRoy Medical Library (Providence Hospital and Medical Centers), http://www.providence-hospital.org/library/

- **Michigan:** Marquette General Hospital - Consumer Health Library (Marquette General Hospital, Health Information Center), http://www.mgh.org/center.html

- **Michigan:** Patient Education Resouce Center - University of Michigan Cancer Center (University of Michigan Comprehensive Cancer Center, Ann Arbor), http://www.cancer.med.umich.edu/learn/leares.htm

- **Michigan:** Sladen Library & Center for Health Information Resources - Consumer Health Information (Detroit), http://www.henryford.com/body.cfm?id=39330

- **Montana:** Center for Health Information (St. Patrick Hospital and Health Sciences Center, Missoula)

- **National:** Consumer Health Library Directory (Medical Library Association, Consumer and Patient Health Information Section), http://caphis.mlanet.org/directory/index.html

- **National:** National Network of Libraries of Medicine (National Library of Medicine) - provides library services for health professionals in the United States who do not have access to a medical library, http://nnlm.gov/

- **National:** NN/LM List of Libraries Serving the Public (National Network of Libraries of Medicine), http://nnlm.gov/members/

- **Nevada:** Health Science Library, West Charleston Library (Las Vegas-Clark County Library District, Las Vegas), **http://www.lvccld.org/special_collections/medical/index.htm**

- **New Hampshire:** Dartmouth Biomedical Libraries (Dartmouth College Library, Hanover), **http://www.dartmouth.edu/~biomed/resources.htmld/conshealth.htmld/**

- **New Jersey:** Consumer Health Library (Rahway Hospital, Rahway), **http://www.rahwayhospital.com/library.htm**

- **New Jersey:** Dr. Walter Phillips Health Sciences Library (Englewood Hospital and Medical Center, Englewood), **http://www.englewoodhospital.com/links/index.htm**

- **New Jersey:** Meland Foundation (Englewood Hospital and Medical Center, Englewood), **http://www.geocities.com/ResearchTriangle/9360/**

- **New York:** Choices in Health Information (New York Public Library) - NLM Consumer Pilot Project participant, **http://www.nypl.org/branch/health/links.html**

- **New York:** Health Information Center (Upstate Medical University, State University of New York, Syracuse), **http://www.upstate.edu/library/hic/**

- **New York:** Health Sciences Library (Long Island Jewish Medical Center, New Hyde Park), **http://www.lij.edu/library/library.html**

- **New York:** ViaHealth Medical Library (Rochester General Hospital), **http://www.nyam.org/library/**

- **Ohio:** Consumer Health Library (Akron General Medical Center, Medical & Consumer Health Library), **http://www.akrongeneral.org/hwlibrary.htm**

- **Oklahoma:** The Health Information Center at Saint Francis Hospital (Saint Francis Health System, Tulsa), **http://www.sfh-tulsa.com/services/healthinfo.asp**

- **Oregon:** Planetree Health Resource Center (Mid-Columbia Medical Center, The Dalles), **http://www.mcmc.net/phrc/**

- **Pennsylvania:** Community Health Information Library (Milton S. Hershey Medical Center, Hershey), **http://www.hmc.psu.edu/commhealth/**

- **Pennsylvania:** Community Health Resource Library (Geisinger Medical Center, Danville), **http://www.geisinger.edu/education/commlib.shtml**

- **Pennsylvania:** HealthInfo Library (Moses Taylor Hospital, Scranton), **http://www.mth.org/healthwellness.html**

- **Pennsylvania:** Hopwood Library (University of Pittsburgh, Health Sciences Library System, Pittsburgh), **http://www.hsls.pitt.edu/guides/chi/hopwood/index_html**

- **Pennsylvania:** Koop Community Health Information Center (College of Physicians of Philadelphia), **http://www.collphyphil.org/kooppg1.shtml**

- **Pennsylvania:** Learning Resources Center - Medical Library (Susquehanna Health System, Williamsport), **http://www.shscares.org/services/lrc/index.asp**

- **Pennsylvania:** Medical Library (UPMC Health System, Pittsburgh), **http://www.upmc.edu/passavant/library.htm**

- **Quebec, Canada:** Medical Library (Montreal General Hospital), **http://www.mghlib.mcgill.ca/**

- **South Dakota:** Rapid City Regional Hospital Medical Library (Rapid City Regional Hospital), **http://www.rcrh.org/Services/Library/Default.asp**

- **Texas:** Houston HealthWays (Houston Academy of Medicine-Texas Medical Center Library), **http://hhw.library.tmc.edu/**

- **Washington:** Community Health Library (Kittitas Valley Community Hospital), **http://www.kvch.com/**

- **Washington:** Southwest Washington Medical Center Library (Southwest Washington Medical Center, Vancouver), **http://www.swmedicalcenter.com/body.cfm?id=72**

ONLINE GLOSSARIES

The Internet provides access to a number of free-to-use medical dictionaries. The National Library of Medicine has compiled the following list of online dictionaries:

- ADAM Medical Encyclopedia (A.D.A.M., Inc.), comprehensive medical reference: **http://www.nlm.nih.gov/medlineplus/encyclopedia.html**

- MedicineNet.com Medical Dictionary (MedicineNet, Inc.): **http://www.medterms.com/Script/Main/hp.asp**

- Merriam-Webster Medical Dictionary (Inteli-Health, Inc.): **http://www.intelihealth.com/IH/**

- Multilingual Glossary of Technical and Popular Medical Terms in Eight European Languages (European Commission) - Danish, Dutch, English, French, German, Italian, Portuguese, and Spanish: **http://allserv.rug.ac.be/~rvdstich/eugloss/welcome.html**

- On-line Medical Dictionary (CancerWEB): **http://cancerweb.ncl.ac.uk/omd/**

- Rare Diseases Terms (Office of Rare Diseases): **http://ord.aspensys.com/asp/diseases/diseases.asp**

- Technology Glossary (National Library of Medicine) - Health Care Technology: **http://www.nlm.nih.gov/nichsr/ta101/ta10108.htm**

Beyond these, MEDLINEplus contains a very patient-friendly encyclopedia covering every aspect of medicine (licensed from A.D.A.M., Inc.). The ADAM Medical Encyclopedia can be accessed at **http://www.nlm.nih.gov/medlineplus/encyclopedia.html**. ADAM is also available on commercial Web sites such as drkoop.com (**http://www.drkoop.com/**) and Web MD (**http://my.webmd.com/adam/asset/adam_disease_articles/a_to_z/a**). The NIH suggests the following Web sites in the ADAM Medical Encyclopedia when searching for information on bruxism:

- **Basic Guidelines for Bruxism**

  Bruxism
  Web site: http://www.nlm.nih.gov/medlineplus/ency/article/001413.htm

- **Signs & Symptoms for Bruxism**

  Anxiety
  Web site: http://www.nlm.nih.gov/medlineplus/ency/article/003211.htm

  Anxiety, stress, and tension
  Web site: http://www.nlm.nih.gov/medlineplus/ency/article/003211.htm

  Ear pain
  Web site: http://www.nlm.nih.gov/medlineplus/ency/article/003046.htm

  Earache
  Web site: http://www.nlm.nih.gov/medlineplus/ency/article/003046.htm

Muscle
Web site: http://www.nlm.nih.gov/medlineplus/ency/article/003193.htm

Stress
Web site: http://www.nlm.nih.gov/medlineplus/ency/article/003211.htm

Tension
Web site: http://www.nlm.nih.gov/medlineplus/ency/article/003211.htm

- **Background Topics for Bruxism**

  Alcohol use
  Web site: http://www.nlm.nih.gov/medlineplus/ency/article/001944.htm

  Stress management
  Web site: http://www.nlm.nih.gov/medlineplus/ency/article/001942.htm

Online Dictionary Directories

The following are additional online directories compiled by the National Library of Medicine, including a number of specialized medical dictionaries:

- Medical Dictionaries: Medical & Biological (World Health Organization):
  http://www.who.int/hlt/virtuallibrary/English/diction.htm#Medical

- MEL-Michigan Electronic Library List of Online Health and Medical Dictionaries (Michigan Electronic Library): **http://mel.lib.mi.us/health/health-dictionaries.html**

- Patient Education: Glossaries (DMOZ Open Directory Project):
  http://dmoz.org/Health/Education/Patient_Education/Glossaries/

- Web of Online Dictionaries (Bucknell University):
  http://www.yourdictionary.com/diction5.html#medicine

BRUXISM DICTIONARY

The definitions below are derived from official public sources, including the National Institutes of Health [NIH] and the European Union [EU].

Accommodation: Adjustment, especially that of the eye for various distances. [EU]

Action Potentials: The electric response of a nerve or muscle to its stimulation. [NIH]

Acupuncture Analgesia: Analgesia produced by the insertion of acupuncture needles at certain points in the body. These activate the small myelinated nerve fibers in the muscle which transmit impulses to the spinal cord and then activate three centers - the spinal cord, midbrain and pituitary hypothalamus - to produce analgesia. [NIH]

Adjustment: The dynamic process wherein the thoughts, feelings, behavior, and biophysiological mechanisms of the individual continually change to adjust to the environment. [NIH]

Adrenal Medulla: The inner part of the adrenal gland; it synthesizes, stores and releases catecholamines. [NIH]

Adrenergic: Activated by, characteristic of, or secreting epinephrine or substances with similar activity; the term is applied to those nerve fibres that liberate norepinephrine at a synapse when a nerve impulse passes, i.e., the sympathetic fibres. [EU]

Adverse Effect: An unwanted side effect of treatment. [NIH]

Aetiology: Study of the causes of disease. [EU]

Afferent: Concerned with the transmission of neural impulse toward the central part of the nervous system. [NIH]

Affinity: 1. Inherent likeness or relationship. 2. A special attraction for a specific element, organ, or structure. 3. Chemical affinity; the force that binds atoms in molecules; the tendency of substances to combine by chemical reaction. 4. The strength of noncovalent chemical binding between two substances as measured by the dissociation constant of the complex. 5. In immunology, a thermodynamic expression of the strength of interaction between a single antigen-binding site and a single antigenic determinant (and thus of the stereochemical compatibility between them), most accurately applied to interactions among simple, uniform antigenic determinants such as haptens. Expressed as the association constant (K litres mole -1), which, owing to the heterogeneity of affinities in a population of antibody molecules of a given specificity, actually represents an average value (mean intrinsic association constant). 6. The reciprocal of the dissociation constant. [EU]

Agar: A complex sulfated polymer of galactose units, extracted from Gelidium cartilagineum, Gracilaria confervoides, and related red algae. It is used as a gel in the preparation of solid culture media for microorganisms, as a bulk laxative, in making emulsions, and as a supporting medium for immunodiffusion and immunoelectrophoresis. [NIH]

Agonist: In anatomy, a prime mover. In pharmacology, a drug that has affinity for and stimulates physiologic activity at cell receptors normally stimulated by naturally occurring substances. [EU]

Airway: A device for securing unobstructed passage of air into and out of the lungs during general anesthesia. [NIH]

Airway Obstruction: Any hindrance to the passage of air into and out of the lungs. [NIH]

Akathisia: 1. A condition of motor restlessness in which there is a feeling of muscular quivering, an urge to move about constantly, and an inability to sit still, a common extrapyramidal side effect of neuroleptic drugs. 2. An inability to sit down because of intense anxiety at the thought of doing so. [EU]

Algorithms: A procedure consisting of a sequence of algebraic formulas and/or logical steps to calculate or determine a given task. [NIH]

Alkaline: Having the reactions of an alkali. [EU]

Alkaloid: A member of a large group of chemicals that are made by plants and have nitrogen in them. Some alkaloids have been shown to work against cancer. [NIH]

Alpha-1: A protein with the property of inactivating proteolytic enzymes such as leucocyte collagenase and elastase. [NIH]

Alternative medicine: Practices not generally recognized by the medical community as standard or conventional medical approaches and used instead of standard treatments. Alternative medicine includes the taking of dietary supplements, megadose vitamins, and herbal preparations; the drinking of special teas; and practices such as massage therapy, magnet therapy, spiritual healing, and meditation. [NIH]

Alveolar Process: The thickest and spongiest part of the maxilla and mandible hollowed out into deep cavities for the teeth. [NIH]

Alveoli: Tiny air sacs at the end of the bronchioles in the lungs. [NIH]

Amenorrhea: Absence of menstruation. [NIH]

Amitriptyline: Tricyclic antidepressant with anticholinergic and sedative properties. It appears to prevent the re-uptake of norepinephrine and serotonin at nerve terminals, thus potentiating the action of these neurotransmitters. Amitriptyline also appears to antaganize cholinergic and alpha-1 adrenergic responses to bioactive amines. [NIH]

Amnestic: Nominal aphasia; a difficulty in finding the right name for an object. [NIH]

Anaesthesia: Loss of feeling or sensation. Although the term is used for loss of tactile sensibility, or of any of the other senses, it is applied especially to loss of the sensation of pain, as it is induced to permit performance of surgery or other painful procedures. [EU]

Anal: Having to do with the anus, which is the posterior opening of the large bowel. [NIH]

Analgesic: An agent that alleviates pain without causing loss of consciousness. [EU]

Anaphylatoxins: The family of peptides C3a, C4a, C5a, and C5a des-arginine produced in the serum during complement activation. They produce smooth muscle contraction, mast cell histamine release, affect platelet aggregation, and act as mediators of the local inflammatory process. The order of anaphylatoxin activity from strongest to weakest is C5a, C3a, C4a, and C5a des-arginine. The latter is the so-called "classical" anaphylatoxin but shows no spasmogenic activity though it contains some chemotactic ability. [NIH]

Anatomical: Pertaining to anatomy, or to the structure of the organism. [EU]

Anesthesia: A state characterized by loss of feeling or sensation. This depression of nerve function is usually the result of pharmacologic action and is induced to allow performance of surgery or other painful procedures. [NIH]

Angina: Chest pain that originates in the heart. [NIH]

Angina Pectoris: The symptom of paroxysmal pain consequent to myocardial ischemia usually of distinctive character, location and radiation, and provoked by a transient stressful situation during which the oxygen requirements of the myocardium exceed the capacity of the coronary circulation to supply it. [NIH]

Anomalies: Birth defects; abnormalities. [NIH]

Antibody: A type of protein made by certain white blood cells in response to a foreign substance (antigen). Each antibody can bind to only a specific antigen. The purpose of this binding is to help destroy the antigen. Antibodies can work in several ways, depending on the nature of the antigen. Some antibodies destroy antigens directly. Others make it easier for white blood cells to destroy the antigen. [NIH]

Anticholinergic: An agent that blocks the parasympathetic nerves. Called also parasympatholytic. [EU]

Anticonvulsant: An agent that prevents or relieves convulsions. [EU]

Antidepressant: A drug used to treat depression. [NIH]

Antidopaminergic: Preventing or counteracting (the effects of) dopamine. [EU]

Antidote: A remedy for counteracting a poison. [EU]

Antiemetic: An agent that prevents or alleviates nausea and vomiting. Also antinauseant. [EU]

Antigen: Any substance which is capable, under appropriate conditions, of inducing a specific immune response and of reacting with the products of that response, that is, with specific antibody or specifically sensitized T-lymphocytes, or both. Antigens may be soluble substances, such as toxins and foreign proteins, or particulate, such as bacteria and tissue cells; however, only the portion of the protein or polysaccharide molecule known as the antigenic determinant (q.v.) combines with antibody or a specific receptor on a lymphocyte. Abbreviated Ag. [EU]

Antigen-Antibody Complex: The complex formed by the binding of antigen and antibody molecules. The deposition of large antigen-antibody complexes leading to tissue damage causes immune complex diseases. [NIH]

Anti-infective: An agent that so acts. [EU]

Anti-inflammatory: Having to do with reducing inflammation. [NIH]

Antipsychotic: Effective in the treatment of psychosis. Antipsychotic drugs (called also neuroleptic drugs and major tranquilizers) are a chemically diverse (including phenothiazines, thioxanthenes, butyrophenones, dibenzoxazepines, dibenzodiazepines, and diphenylbutylpiperidines) but pharmacologically similar class of drugs used to treat schizophrenic, paranoid, schizoaffective, and other psychotic disorders; acute delirium and dementia, and manic episodes (during induction of lithium therapy); to control the movement disorders associated with Huntington's chorea, Gilles de la Tourette's syndrome, and ballismus; and to treat intractable hiccups and severe nausea and vomiting. Antipsychotic agents bind to dopamine, histamine, muscarinic cholinergic, a-adrenergic, and serotonin receptors. Blockade of dopaminergic transmission in various areas is thought to be responsible for their major effects : antipsychotic action by blockade in the mesolimbic and mesocortical areas; extrapyramidal side effects (dystonia, akathisia, parkinsonism, and tardive dyskinesia) by blockade in the basal ganglia; and antiemetic effects by blockade in the chemoreceptor trigger zone of the medulla. Sedation and autonomic side effects (orthostatic hypotension, blurred vision, dry mouth, nasal congestion and constipation) are caused by blockade of histamine, cholinergic, and adrenergic receptors. [EU]

Antipyretic: An agent that relieves or reduces fever. Called also antifebrile, antithermic and febrifuge. [EU]

Anus: The opening of the rectum to the outside of the body. [NIH]

Anxiety: Persistent feeling of dread, apprehension, and impending disaster. [NIH]

Aphthous Stomatitis: Inflammation of the mucous membrane of the mouth. [NIH]

Apnea: A transient absence of spontaneous respiration. [NIH]

Aponeurosis: Tendinous expansion consisting of a fibrous or membranous sheath which serves as a fascia to enclose or bind a group of muscles. [NIH]

Artery: Vessel-carrying blood from the heart to various parts of the body. [NIH]

Articular: Of or pertaining to a joint. [EU]

Articulation: The relationship of two bodies by means of a moveable joint. [NIH]

Astringents: Agents, usually topical, that cause the contraction of tissues for the control of bleeding or secretions. [NIH]

Astrocytes: The largest and most numerous neuroglial cells in the brain and spinal cord. Astrocytes (from "star" cells) are irregularly shaped with many long processes, including those with "end feet" which form the glial (limiting) membrane and directly and indirectly contribute to the blood brain barrier. They regulate the extracellular ionic and chemical environment, and "reactive astrocytes" (along with microglia) respond to injury. Astrocytes have high- affinity transmitter uptake systems, voltage-dependent and transmitter-gated ion channels, and can release transmitter, but their role in signaling (as in many other functions) is not well understood. [NIH]

Autoimmune disease: A condition in which the body recognizes its own tissues as foreign and directs an immune response against them. [NIH]

Axons: Nerve fibers that are capable of rapidly conducting impulses away from the neuron cell body. [NIH]

Bacteria: Unicellular prokaryotic microorganisms which generally possess rigid cell walls, multiply by cell division, and exhibit three principal forms: round or coccal, rodlike or bacillary, and spiral or spirochetal. [NIH]

Basal Ganglia: Large subcortical nuclear masses derived from the telencephalon and located in the basal regions of the cerebral hemispheres. [NIH]

Base: In chemistry, the nonacid part of a salt; a substance that combines with acids to form salts; a substance that dissociates to give hydroxide ions in aqueous solutions; a substance whose molecule or ion can combine with a proton (hydrogen ion); a substance capable of donating a pair of electrons (to an acid) for the formation of a coordinate covalent bond. [EU]

Benign: Not cancerous; does not invade nearby tissue or spread to other parts of the body. [NIH]

Bewilderment: Impairment or loss of will power. [NIH]

Bilateral: Affecting both the right and left side of body. [NIH]

Bile: An emulsifying agent produced in the liver and secreted into the duodenum. Its composition includes bile acids and salts, cholesterol, and electrolytes. It aids digestion of fats in the duodenum. [NIH]

Bile Acids: Acids made by the liver that work with bile to break down fats. [NIH]

Biochemical: Relating to biochemistry; characterized by, produced by, or involving chemical reactions in living organisms. [EU]

Biopsy: Removal and pathologic examination of specimens in the form of small pieces of tissue from the living body. [NIH]

Biotechnology: Body of knowledge related to the use of organisms, cells or cell-derived constituents for the purpose of developing products which are technically, scientifically and clinically useful. Alteration of biologic function at the molecular level (i.e., genetic engineering) is a central focus; laboratory methods used include transfection and cloning technologies, sequence and structure analysis algorithms, computer databases, and gene and protein structure function analysis and prediction. [NIH]

Biotransformation: The chemical alteration of an exogenous substance by or in a biological system. The alteration may inactivate the compound or it may result in the production of an active metabolite of an inactive parent compound. The alteration may be either non-synthetic (oxidation-reduction, hydrolysis) or synthetic (glucuronide formation, sulfate conjugation, acetylation, methylation). This also includes metabolic detoxication and clearance. [NIH]

Bite Force: The force applied by the masticatory muscles in dental occlusion. [NIH]

Bladder: The organ that stores urine. [NIH]

Blood Coagulation: The process of the interaction of blood coagulation factors that results in an insoluble fibrin clot. [NIH]

Blood Platelets: Non-nucleated disk-shaped cells formed in the megakaryocyte and found in the blood of all mammals. They are mainly involved in blood coagulation. [NIH]

Blood pressure: The pressure of blood against the walls of a blood vessel or heart chamber. Unless there is reference to another location, such as the pulmonary artery or one of the heart chambers, it refers to the pressure in the systemic arteries, as measured, for example, in the forearm. [NIH]

Blood vessel: A tube in the body through which blood circulates. Blood vessels include a network of arteries, arterioles, capillaries, venules, and veins. [NIH]

Bone Resorption: Bone loss due to osteoclastic activity. [NIH]

Bowel: The long tube-shaped organ in the abdomen that completes the process of digestion. There is both a small and a large bowel. Also called the intestine. [NIH]

Brace: Any form of splint or appliance used to support the limbs or trunk. [NIH]

Brain Stem: The part of the brain that connects the cerebral hemispheres with the spinal cord. It consists of the mesencephalon, pons, and medulla oblongata. [NIH]

Bromocriptine: A semisynthetic ergot alkaloid that is a dopamine D2 agonist. It suppresses prolactin secretion and is used to treat amenorrhea, galactorrhea, and female infertility, and has been proposed for Parkinson disease. [NIH]

Bruxism: A disorder characterized by grinding and clenching of the teeth. [NIH]

Buccal: Pertaining to or directed toward the cheek. In dental anatomy, used to refer to the buccal surface of a tooth. [EU]

Calcium: A basic element found in nearly all organized tissues. It is a member of the alkaline earth family of metals with the atomic symbol Ca, atomic number 20, and atomic weight 40. Calcium is the most abundant mineral in the body and combines with phosphorus to form calcium phosphate in the bones and teeth. It is essential for the normal functioning of nerves and muscles and plays a role in blood coagulation (as factor IV) and in many enzymatic processes. [NIH]

Calcium Pyrophosphate: Diphosphoric acid, calcium salt. An inorganic pyrophosphate which affects calcium metabolism in mammals. Abnormalities in its metabolism occur in some human diseases, notably hypophosphatasia and pseudogout. [NIH]

Candidiasis: Infection with a fungus of the genus Candida. It is usually a superficial infection of the moist cutaneous areas of the body, and is generally caused by C. albicans; it most commonly involves the skin (dermatocandidiasis), oral mucous membranes (thrush, def. 1), respiratory tract (bronchocandidiasis), and vagina (vaginitis). Rarely there is a systemic infection or endocarditis. Called also moniliasis, candidosis, oidiomycosis, and formerly blastodendriosis. [EU]

Candidosis: An infection caused by an opportunistic yeasts that tends to proliferate and become pathologic when the environment is favorable and the host resistance is weakened. [NIH]

Capsules: Hard or soft soluble containers used for the oral administration of medicine. [NIH]

Cardiac: Having to do with the heart. [NIH]

Cardioselective: Having greater activity on heart tissue than on other tissue. [EU]

Cardiovascular: Having to do with the heart and blood vessels. [NIH]

Case report: A detailed report of the diagnosis, treatment, and follow-up of an individual patient. Case reports also contain some demographic information about the patient (for example, age, gender, ethnic origin). [NIH]

Case series: A group or series of case reports involving patients who were given similar treatment. Reports of case series usually contain detailed information about the individual patients. This includes demographic information (for example, age, gender, ethnic origin) and information on diagnosis, treatment, response to treatment, and follow-up after treatment. [NIH]

Catecholamine: A group of chemical substances manufactured by the adrenal medulla and secreted during physiological stress. [NIH]

Caudal: Denoting a position more toward the cauda, or tail, than some specified point of reference; same as inferior, in human anatomy. [EU]

Causal: Pertaining to a cause; directed against a cause. [EU]

Cell: The individual unit that makes up all of the tissues of the body. All living things are made up of one or more cells. [NIH]

Cell membrane: Cell membrane = plasma membrane. The structure enveloping a cell, enclosing the cytoplasm, and forming a selective permeability barrier; it consists of lipids, proteins, and some carbohydrates, the lipids thought to form a bilayer in which integral proteins are embedded to varying degrees. [EU]

Central Nervous System: The main information-processing organs of the nervous system, consisting of the brain, spinal cord, and meninges. [NIH]

Central Nervous System Infections: Pathogenic infections of the brain, spinal cord, and meninges. DNA virus infections; RNA virus infections; bacterial infections; mycoplasma infections; Spirochaetales infections; fungal infections; protozoan infections; helminthiasis; and prion diseases may involve the central nervous system as a primary or secondary process. [NIH]

Centric Relation: The location of the maxillary and the mandibular condyles when they are in their most posterior and superior positions in their fossae of the temporomandibular joint. [NIH]

Cerebellar: Pertaining to the cerebellum. [EU]

Cerebellum: Part of the metencephalon that lies in the posterior cranial fossa behind the brain stem. It is concerned with the coordination of movement. [NIH]

Cerebral: Of or pertaining of the cerebrum or the brain. [EU]

Cerebral Aqueduct: Narrow channel in the mesencephalon that connects the third and fourth ventricles. [NIH]

Cerebral Palsy: Refers to a motor disability caused by a brain dysfunction. [NIH]

Cerebrum: The largest part of the brain. It is divided into two hemispheres, or halves, called the cerebral hemispheres. The cerebrum controls muscle functions of the body and also controls speech, emotions, reading, writing, and learning. [NIH]

Cervical: Relating to the neck, or to the neck of any organ or structure. Cervical lymph nodes are located in the neck; cervical cancer refers to cancer of the uterine cervix, which is the lower, narrow end (the "neck") of the uterus. [NIH]

Cervix: The lower, narrow end of the uterus that forms a canal between the uterus and vagina. [NIH]

Chemoreceptor: A receptor adapted for excitation by chemical substances, e.g., olfactory and gustatory receptors, or a sense organ, as the carotid body or the aortic (supracardial) bodies, which is sensitive to chemical changes in the blood stream, especially reduced oxygen content, and reflexly increases both respiration and blood pressure. [EU]

Chemotactic Factors: Chemical substances that attract or repel cells or organisms. The concept denotes especially those factors released as a result of tissue injury, invasion, or immunologic activity, that attract leukocytes, macrophages, or other cells to the site of infection or insult. [NIH]

Chemotherapeutic agent: A drug used to treat cancer. [NIH]

Chin: The anatomical frontal portion of the mandible, also known as the mentum, that contains the line of fusion of the two separate halves of the mandible (symphysis menti). This line of fusion divides inferiorly to enclose a triangular area called the mental protuberance. On each side, inferior to the second premolar tooth, is the mental foramen for the passage of blood vessels and a nerve. [NIH]

Cholinergic: Resembling acetylcholine in pharmacological action; stimulated by or releasing acetylcholine or a related compound. [EU]

Chorea: Involuntary, forcible, rapid, jerky movements that may be subtle or become confluent, markedly altering normal patterns of movement. Hypotonia and pendular reflexes are often associated. Conditions which feature recurrent or persistent episodes of chorea as a primary manifestation of disease are referred to as choreatic disorders. Chorea is also a frequent manifestation of basal ganglia diseases. [NIH]

Chronic: A disease or condition that persists or progresses over a long period of time. [NIH]

Clamp: A u-shaped steel rod used with a pin or wire for skeletal traction in the treatment of certain fractures. [NIH]

Clinical Medicine: The study and practice of medicine by direct examination of the patient. [NIH]

Clinical study: A research study in which patients receive treatment in a clinic or other medical facility. Reports of clinical studies can contain results for single patients (case reports) or many patients (case series or clinical trials). [NIH]

Clinical trial: A research study that tests how well new medical treatments or other interventions work in people. Each study is designed to test new methods of screening, prevention, diagnosis, or treatment of a disease. [NIH]

Cloning: The production of a number of genetically identical individuals; in genetic engineering, a process for the efficient replication of a great number of identical DNA molecules. [NIH]

Cochlea: The part of the internal ear that is concerned with hearing. It forms the anterior part of the labyrinth, is conical, and is placed almost horizontally anterior to the vestibule. [NIH]

Collapse: 1. A state of extreme prostration and depression, with failure of circulation. 2. Abnormal falling in of the walls of any part of organ. [EU]

Complement: A term originally used to refer to the heat-labile factor in serum that causes immune cytolysis, the lysis of antibody-coated cells, and now referring to the entire functionally related system comprising at least 20 distinct serum proteins that is the effector not only of immune cytolysis but also of other biologic functions. Complement activation occurs by two different sequences, the classic and alternative pathways. The proteins of the classic pathway are termed 'components of complement' and are designated by the symbols C1 through C9. C1 is a calcium-dependent complex of three distinct proteins C1q, C1r and C1s. The proteins of the alternative pathway (collectively referred to as the properdin system) and complement regulatory proteins are known by semisystematic or trivial names. Fragments resulting from proteolytic cleavage of complement proteins are designated with lower-case letter suffixes, e.g., C3a. Inactivated fragments may be designated with the suffix 'i', e.g. C3bi. Activated components or complexes with biological activity are designated by a bar over the symbol e.g. C1 or C4b,2a. The classic pathway is activated by the binding of C1 to classic pathway activators, primarily antigen-antibody complexes containing IgM, IgG1, IgG3; C1q binds to a single IgM molecule or two adjacent IgG molecules. The alternative pathway can be activated by IgA immune complexes and also by nonimmunologic materials including bacterial endotoxins, microbial polysaccharides, and cell walls. Activation of the classic pathway triggers an enzymatic cascade involving C1, C4, C2 and C3; activation of the alternative pathway triggers a cascade involving C3 and factors B, D and P. Both result in the cleavage of C5 and the formation of the membrane attack complex. Complement activation also results in the formation of many biologically active complement fragments that act as anaphylatoxins, opsonins, or chemotactic factors. [EU]

Complementary and alternative medicine: CAM. Forms of treatment that are used in addition to (complementary) or instead of (alternative) standard treatments. These practices are not considered standard medical approaches. CAM includes dietary supplements, megadose vitamins, herbal preparations, special teas, massage therapy, magnet therapy, spiritual healing, and meditation. [NIH]

Complementary medicine: Practices not generally recognized by the medical community as standard or conventional medical approaches and used to enhance or complement the standard treatments. Complementary medicine includes the taking of dietary supplements, megadose vitamins, and herbal preparations; the drinking of special teas; and practices such as massage therapy, magnet therapy, spiritual healing, and meditation. [NIH]

Computational Biology: A field of biology concerned with the development of techniques for the collection and manipulation of biological data, and the use of such data to make biological discoveries or predictions. This field encompasses all computational methods and theories applicable to molecular biology and areas of computer-based techniques for solving biological problems including manipulation of models and datasets. [NIH]

Computed tomography: CT scan. A series of detailed pictures of areas inside the body, taken from different angles; the pictures are created by a computer linked to an x-ray machine. Also called computerized tomography and computerized axial tomography (CAT) scan. [NIH]

Computerized axial tomography: A series of detailed pictures of areas inside the body, taken from different angles; the pictures are created by a computer linked to an x-ray machine. Also called CAT scan, computed tomography (CT scan), or computerized tomography. [NIH]

Computerized tomography: A series of detailed pictures of areas inside the body, taken from different angles; the pictures are created by a computer linked to an x-ray machine. Also called computerized axial tomography (CAT) scan and computed tomography (CT scan). [NIH]

Concomitant: Accompanying; accessory; joined with another. [EU]

Conduction: The transfer of sound waves, heat, nervous impulses, or electricity. [EU]

Confusion: A mental state characterized by bewilderment, emotional disturbance, lack of clear thinking, and perceptual disorientation. [NIH]

Congestion: Excessive or abnormal accumulation of blood in a part. [EU]

Conjugation: 1. The act of joining together or the state of being conjugated. 2. A sexual process seen in bacteria, ciliate protozoa, and certain fungi in which nuclear material is exchanged during the temporary fusion of two cells (conjugants). In bacterial genetics a form of sexual reproduction in which a donor bacterium (male) contributes some, or all, of its DNA (in the form of a replicated set) to a recipient (female) which then incorporates differing genetic information into its own chromosome by recombination and passes the recombined set on to its progeny by replication. In ciliate protozoa, two conjugants of separate mating types exchange micronuclear material and then separate, each now being a fertilized cell. In certain fungi, the process involves fusion of two gametes, resulting in union of their nuclei and formation of a zygote. 3. In chemistry, the joining together of two compounds to produce another compound, such as the combination of a toxic product with some substance in the body to form a detoxified product, which is then eliminated. [EU]

Conjunctiva: The mucous membrane that lines the inner surface of the eyelids and the anterior part of the sclera. [NIH]

Consciousness: Sense of awareness of self and of the environment. [NIH]

Constipation: Infrequent or difficult evacuation of feces. [NIH]

Contraindications: Any factor or sign that it is unwise to pursue a certain kind of action or treatment, e. g. giving a general anesthetic to a person with pneumonia. [NIH]

Contralateral: Having to do with the opposite side of the body. [NIH]

Controlled clinical trial: A clinical study that includes a comparison (control) group. The comparison group receives a placebo, another treatment, or no treatment at all. [NIH]

Controlled study: An experiment or clinical trial that includes a comparison (control) group. [NIH]

Convulsions: A general term referring to sudden and often violent motor activity of cerebral or brainstem origin. Convulsions may also occur in the absence of an electrical cerebral discharge (e.g., in response to hypotension). [NIH]

Coordination: Muscular or motor regulation or the harmonious cooperation of muscles or groups of muscles, in a complex action or series of actions. [NIH]

Cortical: Pertaining to or of the nature of a cortex or bark. [EU]

Cranial: Pertaining to the cranium, or to the anterior (in animals) or superior (in humans) end of the body. [EU]

Craniocerebral Trauma: Traumatic injuries involving the cranium and intracranial structures (i.e., brain; cranial nerves; meninges; and other structures). Injuries may be classified by whether or not the skull is penetrated (i.e., penetrating vs. nonpenetrating) or whether there is an associated hemorrhage. [NIH]

Craniomandibular Disorders: Diseases or disorders of the muscles of the head and neck, with special reference to the masticatory muscles. The most notable examples are temporomandibular joint disorders and temporomandibular joint dysfunction syndrome. [NIH]

Crowding: Behavior with respect to an excessive number of individuals, human or animal, in relation to available space. [NIH]

Curare: Plant extracts from several species, including Strychnos toxifera, S. castelnaei, S. crevauxii, and Chondodendron tomentosum, that produce paralysis of skeletal muscle and are used adjunctively with general anesthesia. These extracts are toxic and must be used with the administration of artificial respiration. [NIH]

Curative: Tending to overcome disease and promote recovery. [EU]

Cutaneous: Having to do with the skin. [NIH]

Degenerative: Undergoing degeneration : tending to degenerate; having the character of or involving degeneration; causing or tending to cause degeneration. [EU]

Deglutition: The process or the act of swallowing. [NIH]

Delirium: (DSM III-R) an acute, reversible organic mental disorder characterized by reduced ability to maintain attention to external stimuli and disorganized thinking as manifested by rambling, irrelevant, or incoherent speech; there are also a reduced level of consciousness, sensory misperceptions, disturbance of the sleep-wakefulness cycle and level of psychomotor activity, disorientation to time, place, or person, and memory impairment. Delirium may be caused by a large number of conditions resulting in derangement of cerebral metabolism, including systemic infection, poisoning, drug intoxication or withdrawal, seizures or head trauma, and metabolic disturbances such as hypoxia, hypoglycaemia, fluid, electrolyte, or acid-base imbalances, or hepatic or renal failure. Called also acute confusional state and acute brain syndrome. [EU]

Dementia: An acquired organic mental disorder with loss of intellectual abilities of sufficient severity to interfere with social or occupational functioning. The dysfunction is multifaceted and involves memory, behavior, personality, judgment, attention, spatial relations, language, abstract thought, and other executive functions. The intellectual decline is usually progressive, and initially spares the level of consciousness. [NIH]

Dendrites: Extensions of the nerve cell body. They are short and branched and receive stimuli from other neurons. [NIH]

Dental Amalgam: An alloy used in restorative dentistry that contains mercury, silver, tin, copper, and possibly zinc. [NIH]

Dental Care: The total of dental diagnostic, preventive, and restorative services provided to meet the needs of a patient (from Illustrated Dictionary of Dentistry, 1982). [NIH]

Dental implant: A small metal pin placed inside the jawbone to mimic the root of a tooth. Dental implants can be used to help anchor a false tooth or teeth, or a crown or bridge. [NIH]

Dentists: Individuals licensed to practice dentistry. [NIH]

Dentition: The teeth in the dental arch; ordinarily used to designate the natural teeth in position in their alveoli. [EU]

Depolarization: The process or act of neutralizing polarity. In neurophysiology, the reversal of the resting potential in excitable cell membranes when stimulated, i.e., the tendency of the cell membrane potential to become positive with respect to the potential outside the cell. [EU]

Dermatoglyphics: The study of the patterns of ridges of the skin of the fingers, palms, toes, and soles. [NIH]

Diagnostic procedure: A method used to identify a disease. [NIH]

Diarrhea: Passage of excessively liquid or excessively frequent stools. [NIH]

Dilator: A device used to stretch or enlarge an opening. [NIH]

Direct: 1. Straight; in a straight line. 2. Performed immediately and without the intervention of subsidiary means. [EU]

Discrete: Made up of separate parts or characterized by lesions which do not become blended; not running together; separate. [NIH]

Disorientation: The loss of proper bearings, or a state of mental confusion as to time, place, or identity. [EU]

Distal: Remote; farther from any point of reference; opposed to proximal. In dentistry, used to designate a position on the dental arch farther from the median line of the jaw. [EU]

Diurnal: Occurring during the day. [EU]

Dizziness: An imprecise term which may refer to a sense of spatial disorientation, motion of the environment, or lightheadedness. [NIH]

Dopa: The racemic or DL form of DOPA, an amino acid found in various legumes. The dextro form has little physiologic activity but the levo form (levodopa) is a very important physiologic mediator and precursor and pharmacological agent. [NIH]

Dopamine: An endogenous catecholamine and prominent neurotransmitter in several systems of the brain. In the synthesis of catecholamines from tyrosine, it is the immediate precursor to norepinephrine and epinephrine. Dopamine is a major transmitter in the extrapyramidal system of the brain, and important in regulating movement. A family of dopaminergic receptor subtypes mediate its action. Dopamine is used pharmacologically for its direct (beta adrenergic agonist) and indirect (adrenergic releasing) sympathomimetic effects including its actions as an inotropic agent and as a renal vasodilator. [NIH]

Dorsal: 1. Pertaining to the back or to any dorsum. 2. Denoting a position more toward the back surface than some other object of reference; same as posterior in human anatomy; superior in the anatomy of quadrupeds. [EU]

Dorsum: A plate of bone which forms the posterior boundary of the sella turcica. [NIH]

Double-blind: Pertaining to a clinical trial or other experiment in which neither the subject nor the person administering treatment knows which treatment any particular subject is receiving. [EU]

Drug Interactions: The action of a drug that may affect the activity, metabolism, or toxicity of another drug. [NIH]

Duct: A tube through which body fluids pass. [NIH]

Dyskinesia: Impairment of the power of voluntary movement, resulting in fragmentary or incomplete movements. [EU]

Dysphagia: Difficulty in swallowing. [EU]

Dystonia: Disordered tonicity of muscle. [EU]

Effector: It is often an enzyme that converts an inactive precursor molecule into an active second messenger. [NIH]

Efferent: Nerve fibers which conduct impulses from the central nervous system to muscles and glands. [NIH]

Efficacy: The extent to which a specific intervention, procedure, regimen, or service produces a beneficial result under ideal conditions. Ideally, the determination of efficacy is based on the results of a randomized control trial. [NIH]

Electroconvulsive Therapy: Electrically induced convulsions primarily used in the treatment of severe affective disorders and schizophrenia. [NIH]

Embryo: The prenatal stage of mammalian development characterized by rapid morphological changes and the differentiation of basic structures. [NIH]

Endocarditis: Exudative and proliferative inflammatory alterations of the endocardium, characterized by the presence of vegetations on the surface of the endocardium or in the endocardium itself, and most commonly involving a heart valve, but sometimes affecting the inner lining of the cardiac chambers or the endocardium elsewhere. It may occur as a primary disorder or as a complication of or in association with another disease. [EU]

Endotoxins: Toxins closely associated with the living cytoplasm or cell wall of certain microorganisms, which do not readily diffuse into the culture medium, but are released upon lysis of the cells. [NIH]

Environmental Health: The science of controlling or modifying those conditions, influences, or forces surrounding man which relate to promoting, establishing, and maintaining health. [NIH]

Enzymatic: Phase where enzyme cuts the precursor protein. [NIH]

Enzyme: A protein that speeds up chemical reactions in the body. [NIH]

Epidermal: Pertaining to or resembling epidermis. Called also epidermic or epidermoid. [EU]

Epidermis: Nonvascular layer of the skin. It is made up, from within outward, of five layers: 1) basal layer (stratum basale epidermidis); 2) spinous layer (stratum spinosum epidermidis); 3) granular layer (stratum granulosum epidermidis); 4) clear layer (stratum lucidum epidermidis); and 5) horny layer (stratum corneum epidermidis). [NIH]

Ergot: Cataract due to ergot poisoning caused by eating of rye cereals contaminated by a fungus. [NIH]

Esophagus: The muscular tube through which food passes from the throat to the stomach. [NIH]

Evoke: The electric response recorded from the cerebral cortex after stimulation of a peripheral sense organ. [NIH]

Excitability: Property of a cardiac cell whereby, when the cell is depolarized to a critical level (called threshold), the membrane becomes permeable and a regenerative inward current causes an action potential. [NIH]

Excitation: An act of irritation or stimulation or of responding to a stimulus; the addition of energy, as the excitation of a molecule by absorption of photons. [EU]

Excitatory: When cortical neurons are excited, their output increases and each new input they receive while they are still excited raises their output markedly. [NIH]

Exogenous: Developed or originating outside the organism, as exogenous disease. [EU]

Extensor: A muscle whose contraction tends to straighten a limb; the antagonist of a flexor. [NIH]

Extracellular: Outside a cell or cells. [EU]

Extracellular Space: Interstitial space between cells, occupied by fluid as well as amorphous and fibrous substances. [NIH]

Extrapyramidal: Outside of the pyramidal tracts. [EU]

Facial: Of or pertaining to the face. [EU]

Facial Nerve: The 7th cranial nerve. The facial nerve has two parts, the larger motor root which may be called the facial nerve proper, and the smaller intermediate or sensory root. Together they provide efferent innervation to the muscles of facial expression and to the lacrimal and salivary glands, and convey afferent information for taste from the anterior two-thirds of the tongue and for touch from the external ear. [NIH]

Facial Pain: Pain in the facial region including orofacial pain and craniofacial pain. Associated conditions include local inflammatory and neoplastic disorders and neuralgic syndromes involving the trigeminal, facial, and glossopharyngeal nerves. Conditions which feature recurrent or persistent facial pain as the primary manifestation of disease are referred to as facial pain syndromes. [NIH]

Family Planning: Programs or services designed to assist the family in controlling reproduction by either improving or diminishing fertility. [NIH]

Fat: Total lipids including phospholipids. [NIH]

Fatigue: The state of weariness following a period of exertion, mental or physical, characterized by a decreased capacity for work and reduced efficiency to respond to stimuli. [NIH]

Fibrosis: Any pathological condition where fibrous connective tissue invades any organ, usually as a consequence of inflammation or other injury. [NIH]

Flatus: Gas passed through the rectum. [NIH]

Flexor: Muscles which flex a joint. [NIH]

Fluvoxamine: A selective serotonin reuptake inhibitor. It is effective in the treatment of depression, obsessive-compulsive disorders, anxiety, panic disorders, and alcohol amnestic disorders. [NIH]

Functional Disorders: Disorders such as irritable bowel syndrome. These conditions result from poor nerve and muscle function. Symptoms such as gas, pain, constipation, and diarrhea come back again and again, but there are no signs of disease or damage. Emotional stress can trigger symptoms. Also called motility disorders. [NIH]

Fungus: A general term used to denote a group of eukaryotic protists, including mushrooms, yeasts, rusts, moulds, smuts, etc., which are characterized by the absence of chlorophyll and by the presence of a rigid cell wall composed of chitin, mannans, and sometimes cellulose. They are usually of simple morphological form or show some reversible cellular specialization, such as the formation of pseudoparenchymatous tissue in the fruiting body of a mushroom. The dimorphic fungi grow, according to environmental conditions, as moulds or yeasts. [EU]

Ganglion: 1. A knot, or knotlike mass. 2. A general term for a group of nerve cell bodies located outside the central nervous system; occasionally applied to certain nuclear groups within the brain or spinal cord, e.g. basal ganglia. 3. A benign cystic tumour occurring on a aponeurosis or tendon, as in the wrist or dorsum of the foot; it consists of a thin fibrous capsule enclosing a clear mucinous fluid. [EU]

Gas: Air that comes from normal breakdown of food. The gases are passed out of the body through the rectum (flatus) or the mouth (burp). [NIH]

Gastric: Having to do with the stomach. [NIH]

Gastroesophageal Reflux: Reflux of gastric juice and/or duodenal contents (bile acids, pancreatic juice) into the distal esophagus, commonly due to incompetence of the lower esophageal sphincter. Gastric regurgitation is an extension of this process with entry of fluid into the pharynx or mouth. [NIH]

Gastrointestinal: Refers to the stomach and intestines. [NIH]

Gastrointestinal tract: The stomach and intestines. [NIH]

Gene: The functional and physical unit of heredity passed from parent to offspring. Genes are pieces of DNA, and most genes contain the information for making a specific protein. [NIH]

Generator: Any system incorporating a fixed parent radionuclide from which is produced a daughter radionuclide which is to be removed by elution or by any other method and used in a radiopharmaceutical. [NIH]

Gingivitis: Inflammation of the gingivae. Gingivitis associated with bony changes is referred to as periodontitis. Called also oulitis and ulitis. [EU]

Gland: An organ that produces and releases one or more substances for use in the body. Some glands produce fluids that affect tissues or organs. Others produce hormones or participate in blood production. [NIH]

Glossitis: Inflammation of the tongue. [NIH]

Glossopharyngeal Nerve: The 9th cranial nerve. The glossopharyngeal nerve is a mixed motor and sensory nerve; it conveys somatic and autonomic efferents as well as general, special, and visceral afferents. Among the connections are motor fibers to the stylopharyngeus muscle, parasympathetic fibers to the parotid glands, general and taste afferents from the posterior third of the tongue, the nasopharynx, and the palate, and afferents from baroreceptors and chemoreceptors of the carotid sinus. [NIH]

Glutamate: Excitatory neurotransmitter of the brain. [NIH]

Governing Board: The group in which legal authority is vested for the control of health-related institutions and organizations. [NIH]

Granuloma: A relatively small nodular inflammatory lesion containing grouped mononuclear phagocytes, caused by infectious and noninfectious agents. [NIH]

Headache: Pain in the cranial region that may occur as an isolated and benign symptom or as a manifestation of a wide variety of conditions including subarachnoid hemorrhage; craniocerebral trauma; central nervous system infections; intracranial hypertension; and other disorders. In general, recurrent headaches that are not associated with a primary disease process are referred to as headache disorders (e.g., migraine). [NIH]

Headache Disorders: Common conditions characterized by persistent or recurrent headaches. Headache syndrome classification systems may be based on etiology (e.g., vascular headache, post-traumatic headaches, etc.), temporal pattern (e.g., cluster headache, paroxysmal hemicrania, etc.), and precipitating factors (e.g., cough headache). [NIH]

Hemicrania: An ache or a pain in one side of the head, as in migraine. [NIH]

Hemorrhage: Bleeding or escape of blood from a vessel. [NIH]

Hemostasis: The process which spontaneously arrests the flow of blood from vessels carrying blood under pressure. It is accomplished by contraction of the vessels, adhesion and aggregation of formed blood elements, and the process of blood or plasma coagulation. [NIH]

Hepatic: Refers to the liver. [NIH]

Hereditary: Of, relating to, or denoting factors that can be transmitted genetically from one generation to another. [NIH]

Histamine: 1H-Imidazole-4-ethanamine. A depressor amine derived by enzymatic decarboxylation of histidine. It is a powerful stimulant of gastric secretion, a constrictor of bronchial smooth muscle, a vasodilator, and also a centrally acting neurotransmitter. [NIH]

Homologous: Corresponding in structure, position, origin, etc., as (a) the feathers of a bird and the scales of a fish, (b) antigen and its specific antibody, (c) allelic chromosomes. [EU]

Hormone: A substance in the body that regulates certain organs. Hormones such as gastrin help in breaking down food. Some hormones come from cells in the stomach and small intestine. [NIH]

Hydrogen: The first chemical element in the periodic table. It has the atomic symbol H, atomic number 1, and atomic weight 1. It exists, under normal conditions, as a colorless, odorless, tasteless, diatomic gas. Hydrogen ions are protons. Besides the common H1 isotope, hydrogen exists as the stable isotope deuterium and the unstable, radioactive isotope tritium. [NIH]

Hydrolysis: The process of cleaving a chemical compound by the addition of a molecule of water. [NIH]

Hyperplasia: An increase in the number of cells in a tissue or organ, not due to tumor formation. It differs from hypertrophy, which is an increase in bulk without an increase in the number of cells. [NIH]

Hypertension: Persistently high arterial blood pressure. Currently accepted threshold levels are 140 mm Hg systolic and 90 mm Hg diastolic pressure. [NIH]

Hyperthyroidism: Excessive functional activity of the thyroid gland. [NIH]

Hypnotherapy: Sleeping-cure. [NIH]

Hypnotic: A drug that acts to induce sleep. [EU]

Hypotension: Abnormally low blood pressure. [NIH]

Hypothalamus: Ventral part of the diencephalon extending from the region of the optic chiasm to the caudal border of the mammillary bodies and forming the inferior and lateral walls of the third ventricle. [NIH]

Ibuprofen: A nonsteroidal anti-inflammatory agent with analgesic properties used in the therapy of rheumatism and arthritis. [NIH]

Illusion: A false interpretation of a genuine percept. [NIH]

Impairment: In the context of health experience, an impairment is any loss or abnormality of psychological, physiological, or anatomical structure or function. [NIH]

In vitro: In the laboratory (outside the body). The opposite of in vivo (in the body). [NIH]

In vivo: In the body. The opposite of in vitro (outside the body or in the laboratory). [NIH]

Incompetence: Physical or mental inadequacy or insufficiency. [EU]

Induction: The act or process of inducing or causing to occur, especially the production of a specific morphogenetic effect in the developing embryo through the influence of evocators or organizers, or the production of anaesthesia or unconsciousness by use of appropriate agents. [EU]

Infection: 1. Invasion and multiplication of microorganisms in body tissues, which may be clinically unapparent or result in local cellular injury due to competitive metabolism, toxins, intracellular replication, or antigen-antibody response. The infection may remain localized, subclinical, and temporary if the body's defensive mechanisms are effective. A local infection may persist and spread by extension to become an acute, subacute, or chronic clinical infection or disease state. A local infection may also become systemic when the microorganisms gain access to the lymphatic or vascular system. 2. An infectious disease. [EU]

Infertility: The diminished or absent ability to conceive or produce an offspring while sterility is the complete inability to conceive or produce an offspring. [NIH]

Inflammation: A pathological process characterized by injury or destruction of tissues caused by a variety of cytologic and chemical reactions. It is usually manifested by typical signs of pain, heat, redness, swelling, and loss of function. [NIH]

Inner ear: The labyrinth, comprising the vestibule, cochlea, and semicircular canals. [NIH]

Inorganic: Pertaining to substances not of organic origin. [EU]

Inositol: An isomer of glucose that has traditionally been considered to be a B vitamin although it has an uncertain status as a vitamin and a deficiency syndrome has not been identified in man. (From Martindale, The Extra Pharmacopoeia, 30th ed, p1379) Inositol phospholipids are important in signal transduction. [NIH]

Insulator: Material covering the metal conductor of the lead. It is usually polyurethane or silicone. [NIH]

Interneurons: Most generally any neurons which are not motor or sensory. Interneurons may also refer to neurons whose axons remain within a particular brain region as contrasted with projection neurons which have axons projecting to other brain regions. [NIH]

Intestines: The section of the alimentary canal from the stomach to the anus. It includes the large intestine and small intestine. [NIH]

Intoxication: Poisoning, the state of being poisoned. [EU]

Intracellular: Inside a cell. [NIH]

Intrinsic: Situated entirely within or pertaining exclusively to a part. [EU]

Involuntary: Reaction occurring without intention or volition. [NIH]

Iodine: A nonmetallic element of the halogen group that is represented by the atomic symbol I, atomic number 53, and atomic weight of 126.90. It is a nutritionally essential element, especially important in thyroid hormone synthesis. In solution, it has anti-infective properties and is used topically. [NIH]

Ion Exchange: Reversible chemical reaction between a solid, often an ION exchange resin, and a fluid whereby ions may be exchanged from one substance to another. This technique is used in water purification, in research, and in industry. [NIH]

Ionization: 1. Any process by which a neutral atom gains or loses electrons, thus acquiring a net charge, as the dissociation of a substance in solution into ions or ion production by the passage of radioactive particles. 2. Iontophoresis. [EU]

Ions: An atom or group of atoms that have a positive or negative electric charge due to a gain (negative charge) or loss (positive charge) of one or more electrons. Atoms with a positive charge are known as cations; those with a negative charge are anions. [NIH]

Iontophoresis: Therapeutic introduction of ions of soluble salts into tissues by means of electric current. In medical literature it is commonly used to indicate the process of increasing the penetration of drugs into surface tissues by the application of electric current. It has nothing to do with ion exchange, air ionization nor phonophoresis, none of which requires current. [NIH]

Irritable Bowel Syndrome: A disorder that comes and goes. Nerves that control the muscles in the GI tract are too active. The GI tract becomes sensitive to food, stool, gas, and stress. Causes abdominal pain, bloating, and constipation or diarrhea. Also called spastic colon or mucous colitis. [NIH]

Isometric Contraction: Muscular contractions characterized by increase in tension without change in length. [NIH]

Isotonic: A biological term denoting a solution in which body cells can be bathed without a net flow of water across the semipermeable cell membrane. Also, denoting a solution having the same tonicity as some other solution with which it is compared, such as physiologic salt solution and the blood serum. [EU]

Isotonic Contraction: Muscle contraction with negligible change in the force of contraction but shortening of the distance between the origin and insertion. [NIH]

Kb: A measure of the length of DNA fragments, 1 Kb = 1000 base pairs. The largest DNA fragments are up to 50 kilobases long. [NIH]

Ketoprofen: An ibuprofen-type anti-inflammatory analgesic and antipyretic. It is used in the treatment of rheumatoid arthritis and osteoarthritis. [NIH]

Labile: 1. Gliding; moving from point to point over the surface; unstable; fluctuating. 2. Chemically unstable. [EU]

Labyrinth: The internal ear; the essential part of the organ of hearing. It consists of an osseous and a membranous portion. [NIH]

Laryngeal: Having to do with the larynx. [NIH]

Larynx: An irregularly shaped, musculocartilaginous tubular structure, lined with mucous membrane, located at the top of the trachea and below the root of the tongue and the hyoid bone. It is the essential sphincter guarding the entrance into the trachea and functioning secondarily as the organ of voice. [NIH]

Latent: Phoria which occurs at one distance or another and which usually has no troublesome effect. [NIH]

Lesion: An area of abnormal tissue change. [NIH]

Leukoplakia: A white patch that may develop on mucous membranes such as the cheek, gums, or tongue and may become cancerous. [NIH]

Levo: It is an experimental treatment for heroin addiction that was developed by German scientists around 1948 as an analgesic. Like methadone, it binds with opioid receptors, but it is longer acting. [NIH]

Levodopa: The naturally occurring form of dopa and the immediate precursor of dopamine. Unlike dopamine itself, it can be taken orally and crosses the blood-brain barrier. It is rapidly taken up by dopaminergic neurons and converted to dopamine. It is used for the treatment of parkinsonism and is usually given with agents that inhibit its conversion to dopamine outside of the central nervous system. [NIH]

Lichen Planus: An inflammatory, pruritic disease of the skin and mucous membranes, which can be either generalized or localized. It is characterized by distinctive purplish, flat-topped papules having a predilection for the trunk and flexor surfaces. The lesions may be discrete or coalesce to form plaques. Histologically, there is a "saw-tooth" pattern of epidermal hyperplasia and vacuolar alteration of the basal layer of the epidermis along with an intense upper dermal inflammatory infiltrate composed predominantly of T-cells. Etiology is unknown. [NIH]

Ligament: A band of fibrous tissue that connects bones or cartilages, serving to support and strengthen joints. [EU]

Lip: Either of the two fleshy, full-blooded margins of the mouth. [NIH]

Lipid: Fat. [NIH]

Lithium: An element in the alkali metals family. It has the atomic symbol Li, atomic number 3, and atomic weight 6.94. Salts of lithium are used in treating manic-depressive disorders. [NIH]

Liver: A large, glandular organ located in the upper abdomen. The liver cleanses the blood and aids in digestion by secreting bile. [NIH]

Localized: Cancer which has not metastasized yet. [NIH]

Lower Esophageal Sphincter: The muscle between the esophagus and stomach. When a person swallows, this muscle relaxes to let food pass from the esophagus to the stomach. It stays closed at other times to keep stomach contents from flowing back into the esophagus. [NIH]

Lymph: The almost colorless fluid that travels through the lymphatic system and carries cells that help fight infection and disease. [NIH]

Lymph node: A rounded mass of lymphatic tissue that is surrounded by a capsule of connective tissue. Also known as a lymph gland. Lymph nodes are spread out along lymphatic vessels and contain many lymphocytes, which filter the lymphatic fluid (lymph). [NIH]

Lymphatic: The tissues and organs, including the bone marrow, spleen, thymus, and lymph nodes, that produce and store cells that fight infection and disease. [NIH]

Mandible: The largest and strongest bone of the face constituting the lower jaw. It supports the lower teeth. [NIH]

Mandibular Condyle: The posterior process on the ramus of the mandible composed of two parts: a superior part, the articular portion, and an inferior part, the condylar neck. [NIH]

Mandibular Nerve: A branch of the trigeminal (5th cranial) nerve. The mandibular nerve carries motor fibers to the muscles of mastication and sensory fibers to the teeth and gingivae, the face in the region of the mandible, and parts of the dura. [NIH]

Manic: Affected with mania. [EU]

Mastication: The act and process of chewing and grinding food in the mouth. [NIH]

Masticatory: 1. subserving or pertaining to mastication; affecting the muscles of mastication. 2. a remedy to be chewed but not swallowed. [EU]

Maxillary: Pertaining to the maxilla : the irregularly shaped bone that with its fellow forms the upper jaw. [EU]

Mediate: Indirect; accomplished by the aid of an intervening medium. [EU]

Mediator: An object or substance by which something is mediated, such as (1) a structure of the nervous system that transmits impulses eliciting a specific response; (2) a chemical substance (transmitter substance) that induces activity in an excitable tissue, such as nerve or muscle; or (3) a substance released from cells as the result of the interaction of antigen with antibody or by the action of antigen with a sensitized lymphocyte. [EU]

MEDLINE: An online database of MEDLARS, the computerized bibliographic Medical Literature Analysis and Retrieval System of the National Library of Medicine. [NIH]

Meiosis: A special method of cell division, occurring in maturation of the germ cells, by means of which each daughter nucleus receives half the number of chromosomes characteristic of the somatic cells of the species. [NIH]

Membrane: A very thin layer of tissue that covers a surface. [NIH]

Memory: Complex mental function having four distinct phases: (1) memorizing or learning, (2) retention, (3) recall, and (4) recognition. Clinically, it is usually subdivided into immediate, recent, and remote memory. [NIH]

Meninges: The three membranes that cover and protect the brain and spinal cord. [NIH]

Menopause: Permanent cessation of menstruation. [NIH]

Mental: Pertaining to the mind; psychic. 2. (L. mentum chin) pertaining to the chin. [EU]

Mental Disorders: Psychiatric illness or diseases manifested by breakdowns in the adaptational process expressed primarily as abnormalities of thought, feeling, and behavior producing either distress or impairment of function. [NIH]

Mental Retardation: Refers to sub-average general intellectual functioning which originated during the developmental period and is associated with impairment in adaptive behavior. [NIH]

Mercury: A silver metallic element that exists as a liquid at room temperature. It has the atomic symbol Hg (from hydrargyrum, liquid silver), atomic number 80, and atomic weight 200.59. Mercury is used in many industrial applications and its salts have been employed therapeutically as purgatives, antisyphilitics, disinfectants, and astringents. It can be absorbed through the skin and mucous membranes which leads to mercury poisoning. Because of its toxicity, the clinical use of mercury and mercurials is diminishing. [NIH]

Mesencephalic: Ipsilateral oculomotor paralysis and contralateral tremor, spasm. or choreic movements of the face and limbs. [NIH]

Mesolimbic: Inner brain region governing emotion and drives. [NIH]

Metabolite: Any substance produced by metabolism or by a metabolic process. [EU]

Metabotropic: A glutamate receptor which triggers an increase in production of 2 intracellular messengers: diacylglycerol and inositol 1, 4, 5-triphosphate. [NIH]

Microdialysis: A technique for measuring extracellular concentrations of substances in tissues, usually in vivo, by means of a small probe equipped with a semipermeable membrane. Substances may also be introduced into the extracellular space through the membrane. [NIH]

Microglia: The third type of glial cell, along with astrocytes and oligodendrocytes (which together form the macroglia). Microglia vary in appearance depending on developmental stage, functional state, and anatomical location; subtype terms include ramified, perivascular, ameboid, resting, and activated. Microglia clearly are capable of phagocytosis and play an important role in a wide spectrum of neuropathologies. They have also been suggested to act in several other roles including in secretion (e.g., of cytokines and neural growth factors), in immunological processing (e.g., antigen presentation), and in central nervous system development and remodeling. [NIH]

Micro-organism: An organism which cannot be observed with the naked eye; e. g. unicellular animals, lower algae, lower fungi, bacteria. [NIH]

Microscopy: The application of microscope magnification to the study of materials that cannot be properly seen by the unaided eye. [NIH]

Modeling: A treatment procedure whereby the therapist presents the target behavior which the learner is to imitate and make part of his repertoire. [NIH]

Modification: A change in an organism, or in a process in an organism, that is acquired from its own activity or environment. [NIH]

Molecular: Of, pertaining to, or composed of molecules : a very small mass of matter. [EU]

Molecule: A chemical made up of two or more atoms. The atoms in a molecule can be the same (an oxygen molecule has two oxygen atoms) or different (a water molecule has two hydrogen atoms and one oxygen atom). Biological molecules, such as proteins and DNA, can be made up of many thousands of atoms. [NIH]

Monitor: An apparatus which automatically records such physiological signs as respiration, pulse, and blood pressure in an anesthetized patient or one undergoing surgical or other procedures. [NIH]

Monoamine: Enzyme that breaks down dopamine in the astrocytes and microglia. [NIH]

Mononuclear: A cell with one nucleus. [NIH]

Morphological: Relating to the configuration or the structure of live organs. [NIH]

Morphology: The science of the form and structure of organisms (plants, animals, and other forms of life). [NIH]

Motility: The ability to move spontaneously. [EU]

Motor Activity: The physical activity of an organism as a behavioral phenomenon. [NIH]

Motor nerve: An efferent nerve conveying an impulse that excites muscular contraction. [NIH]

Movement Disorders: Syndromes which feature dyskinesias as a cardinal manifestation of the disease process. Included in this category are degenerative, hereditary, post-infectious, medication-induced, post-inflammatory, and post-traumatic conditions. [NIH]

Mucinous: Containing or resembling mucin, the main compound in mucus. [NIH]

Mucosa: A mucous membrane, or tunica mucosa. [EU]

Multiple sclerosis: A disorder of the central nervous system marked by weakness, numbness, a loss of muscle coordination, and problems with vision, speech, and bladder control. Multiple sclerosis is thought to be an autoimmune disease in which the body's immune system destroys myelin. Myelin is a substance that contains both protein and fat (lipid) and serves as a nerve insulator and helps in the transmission of nerve signals. [NIH]

Muscle Contraction: A process leading to shortening and/or development of tension in muscle tissue. Muscle contraction occurs by a sliding filament mechanism whereby actin filaments slide inward among the myosin filaments. [NIH]

Muscle Fibers: Large single cells, either cylindrical or prismatic in shape, that form the basic unit of muscle tissue. They consist of a soft contractile substance enclosed in a tubular sheath. [NIH]

Muscle relaxant: An agent that specifically aids in reducing muscle tension, as those acting at the polysynaptic neurons of motor nerves (e.g. meprobamate) or at the myoneural junction (curare and related compounds). [EU]

Muscle Spindles: Mechanoreceptors found between skeletal muscle fibers. Muscle spindles are arranged in parallel with muscle fibers and respond to the passive stretch of the muscle, but cease to discharge if the muscle contracts isotonically, thus signaling muscle length. The muscle spindles are the receptors responsible for the stretch or myotactic reflex. [NIH]

Muscle tension: A force in a material tending to produce extension; the state of being stretched. [NIH]

Musculature: The muscular apparatus of the body, or of any part of it. [EU]

Myelin: The fatty substance that covers and protects nerves. [NIH]

Myocardial infarction: Gross necrosis of the myocardium as a result of interruption of the blood supply to the area; it is almost always caused by atherosclerosis of the coronary arteries, upon which coronary thrombosis is usually superimposed. [NIH]

Myoclonus: Involuntary shock-like contractions, irregular in rhythm and amplitude, followed by relaxation, of a muscle or a group of muscles. This condition may be a feature of some central nervous systems diseases (e.g., epilepsy, myoclonic). Nocturnal myoclonus may represent a normal physiologic event or occur as the principal feature of the nocturnal myoclonus syndrome. (From Adams et al., Principles of Neurology, 6th ed, pp102-3). [NIH]

Myosin: Chief protein in muscle and the main constituent of the thick filaments of muscle fibers. In conjunction with actin, it is responsible for the contraction and relaxation of muscles. [NIH]

Nasal Cavity: The proximal portion of the respiratory passages on either side of the nasal septum, lined with ciliated mucosa, extending from the nares to the pharynx. [NIH]

Nausea: An unpleasant sensation in the stomach usually accompanied by the urge to vomit. Common causes are early pregnancy, sea and motion sickness, emotional stress, intense pain, food poisoning, and various enteroviruses. [NIH]

Neck Muscles: The neck muscles consist of the platysma, splenius cervicis, sternocleidomastoid(eus), longus colli, the anterior, medius, and posterior scalenes, digastric(us), stylohyoid(eus), mylohyoid(eus), geniohyoid(eus), sternohyoid(eus), omohyoid(eus), sternothyroid(eus), and thyrohyoid(eus). [NIH]

Neck Pain: Discomfort or more intense forms of pain that are localized to the cervical region. This term generally refers to pain in the posterior or lateral regions of the neck. [NIH]

Nervous System: The entire nerve apparatus composed of the brain, spinal cord, nerves and ganglia. [NIH]

Neural: 1. Pertaining to a nerve or to the nerves. 2. Situated in the region of the spinal axis, as the neutral arch. [EU]

Neuralgia: Intense or aching pain that occurs along the course or distribution of a peripheral or cranial nerve. [NIH]

Neurogenic: Loss of bladder control caused by damage to the nerves controlling the bladder. [NIH]

Neurogenic Inflammation: Inflammation caused by an injurious stimulus of peripheral neurons and resulting in release of neuropeptides which affect vascular permeability and help initiate proinflammatory and immune reactions at the site of injury. [NIH]

Neuroleptic: A term coined to refer to the effects on cognition and behaviour of antipsychotic drugs, which produce a state of apathy, lack of initiative, and limited range of emotion and in psychotic patients cause a reduction in confusion and agitation and normalization of psychomotor activity. [EU]

Neuromuscular: Pertaining to muscles and nerves. [EU]

Neuronal: Pertaining to a neuron or neurons (= conducting cells of the nervous system). [EU]

Neurons: The basic cellular units of nervous tissue. Each neuron consists of a body, an axon, and dendrites. Their purpose is to receive, conduct, and transmit impulses in the nervous system. [NIH]

Neuropeptides: Peptides released by neurons as intercellular messengers. Many neuropeptides are also hormones released by non-neuronal cells. [NIH]

Neurophysiology: The scientific discipline concerned with the physiology of the nervous system. [NIH]

Neurotransmitter: Any of a group of substances that are released on excitation from the axon terminal of a presynaptic neuron of the central or peripheral nervous system and travel across the synaptic cleft to either excite or inhibit the target cell. Among the many substances that have the properties of a neurotransmitter are acetylcholine, norepinephrine, epinephrine, dopamine, glycine, y-aminobutyrate, glutamic acid, substance P, enkephalins, endorphins, and serotonin. [EU]

Norepinephrine: Precursor of epinephrine that is secreted by the adrenal medulla and is a widespread central and autonomic neurotransmitter. Norepinephrine is the principal transmitter of most postganglionic sympathetic fibers and of the diffuse projection system in the brain arising from the locus ceruleus. It is also found in plants and is used pharmacologically as a sympathomimetic. [NIH]

Nuclear: A test of the structure, blood flow, and function of the kidneys. The doctor injects a mildly radioactive solution into an arm vein and uses x-rays to monitor its progress through the kidneys. [NIH]

Nucleus: A body of specialized protoplasm found in nearly all cells and containing the chromosomes. [NIH]

Obsessive-Compulsive Disorder: An anxiety disorder characterized by recurrent, persistent obsessions or compulsions. Obsessions are the intrusive ideas, thoughts, or images that are experienced as senseless or repugnant. Compulsions are repetitive and seemingly purposeful behavior which the individual generally recognizes as senseless and from which the individual does not derive pleasure although it may provide a release from tension. [NIH]

Occlusal Splints: Rigid or flexible appliances that overlay the occlusal surfaces of the teeth. They are used to treat clenching and bruxism and their sequelae, and to provide temporary relief from muscle or temporomandibular joint pain. [NIH]

Oculomotor: Cranial nerve III. It originate from the lower ventral surface of the midbrain and is classified as a motor nerve. [NIH]

Ophthalmic: Pertaining to the eye. [EU]

Optic Chiasm: The X-shaped structure formed by the meeting of the two optic nerves. At the optic chiasm the fibers from the medial part of each retina cross to project to the other side of the brain while the lateral retinal fibers continue on the same side. As a result each half of the brain receives information about the contralateral visual field from both eyes. [NIH]

Oral Health: The optimal state of the mouth and normal functioning of the organs of the mouth without evidence of disease. [NIH]

Oral Hygiene: The practice of personal hygiene of the mouth. It includes the maintenance of oral cleanliness, tissue tone, and general preservation of oral health. [NIH]

Orofacial: Of or relating to the mouth and face. [EU]

Orthodontics: A dental specialty concerned with the prevention and correction of dental and oral anomalies (malocclusion). [NIH]

Orthostatic: Pertaining to or caused by standing erect. [EU]

Osteoarthritis: A progressive, degenerative joint disease, the most common form of arthritis, especially in older persons. The disease is thought to result not from the aging process but from biochemical changes and biomechanical stresses affecting articular cartilage. In the foreign literature it is often called osteoarthrosis deformans. [NIH]

Outpatient: A patient who is not an inmate of a hospital but receives diagnosis or treatment in a clinic or dispensary connected with the hospital. [NIH]

Overcorrection: A complication of refractive surgery where the achieved amount of correction is more than desired. [NIH]

Oxidation: The act of oxidizing or state of being oxidized. Chemically it consists in the increase of positive charges on an atom or the loss of negative charges. Most biological oxidations are accomplished by the removal of a pair of hydrogen atoms (dehydrogenation) from a molecule. Such oxidations must be accompanied by reduction of an acceptor molecule. Univalent o. indicates loss of one electron; divalent o., the loss of two electrons. [EU]

Oxidation-Reduction: A chemical reaction in which an electron is transferred from one molecule to another. The electron-donating molecule is the reducing agent or reductant; the electron-accepting molecule is the oxidizing agent or oxidant. Reducing and oxidizing agents function as conjugate reductant-oxidant pairs or redox pairs (Lehninger, Principles of Biochemistry, 1982, p471). [NIH]

Paediatric: Of or relating to the care and medical treatment of children; belonging to or concerned with paediatrics. [EU]

Palate: The structure that forms the roof of the mouth. It consists of the anterior hard palate and the posterior soft palate. [NIH]

Palliative: 1. Affording relief, but not cure. 2. An alleviating medicine. [EU]

Pancreatic: Having to do with the pancreas. [NIH]

Pancreatic Juice: The fluid containing digestive enzymes secreted by the pancreas in response to food in the duodenum. [NIH]

Panic: A state of extreme acute, intense anxiety and unreasoning fear accompanied by disorganization of personality function. [NIH]

Panic Disorder: A type of anxiety disorder characterized by unexpected panic attacks that last minutes or, rarely, hours. Panic attacks begin with intense apprehension, fear or terror and, often, a feeling of impending doom. Symptoms experienced during a panic attack include dyspnea or sensations of being smothered; dizziness, loss of balance or faintness; choking sensations; palpitations or accelerated heart rate; shakiness; sweating; nausea or other form of abdominal distress; depersonalization or derealization; paresthesias; hot flashes or chills; chest discomfort or pain; fear of dying and fear of not being in control of oneself or going crazy. Agoraphobia may also develop. Similar to other anxiety disorders, it may be inherited as an autosomal dominant trait. [NIH]

Paralysis: Loss of ability to move all or part of the body. [NIH]

Parkinsonism: A group of neurological disorders characterized by hypokinesia, tremor, and muscular rigidity. [EU]

Parotid: The space that contains the parotid gland, the facial nerve, the external carotid artery, and the retromandibular vein. [NIH]

Paroxetine: A serotonin uptake inhibitor that is effective in the treatment of depression. [NIH]

Paroxysmal: Recurring in paroxysms (= spasms or seizures). [EU]

Patch: A piece of material used to cover or protect a wound, an injured part, etc.: a patch over the eye. [NIH]

Pathologic: 1. Indicative of or caused by a morbid condition. 2. Pertaining to pathology (= branch of medicine that treats the essential nature of the disease, especially the structural and functional changes in tissues and organs of the body caused by the disease). [EU]

Pathophysiology: Altered functions in an individual or an organ due to disease. [NIH]

Patient Education: The teaching or training of patients concerning their own health needs. [NIH]

Perception: The ability quickly and accurately to recognize similarities and differences among presented objects, whether these be pairs of words, pairs of number series, or multiple sets of these or other symbols such as geometric figures. [NIH]

Percutaneous: Performed through the skin, as injection of radiopacque material in radiological examination, or the removal of tissue for biopsy accomplished by a needle. [EU]

Periaqueductal Gray: Central gray matter surrounding the cerebral aqueduct in the mesencephalon. Physiologically it is probably involved in rage reactions, the lordosis reflex, feeding responses, bladder tonus, and pain. [NIH]

Periodontal disease: Disease involving the supporting structures of the teeth (as the gums and periodontal membranes). [NIH]

Periodontal disease: Disease involving the supporting structures of the teeth (as the gums and periodontal membranes). [NIH]

Periodontitis: Inflammation of the periodontal membrane; also called periodontitis simplex. [NIH]

PH: The symbol relating the hydrogen ion (H+) concentration or activity of a solution to that of a given standard solution. Numerically the pH is approximately equal to the negative logarithm of H+ concentration expressed in molarity. pH 7 is neutral; above it alkalinity increases and below it acidity increases. [EU]

Pharmacologic: Pertaining to pharmacology or to the properties and reactions of drugs. [EU]

Pharynx: The hollow tube about 5 inches long that starts behind the nose and ends at the top of the trachea (windpipe) and esophagus (the tube that goes to the stomach). [NIH]

Phenytoin: An anticonvulsant that is used in a wide variety of seizures. It is also an anti-arrhythmic and a muscle relaxant. The mechanism of therapeutic action is not clear, although several cellular actions have been described including effects on ion channels, active transport, and general membrane stabilization. The mechanism of its muscle relaxant effect appears to involve a reduction in the sensitivity of muscle spindles to stretch. Phenytoin has been proposed for several other therapeutic uses, but its use has been limited by its many adverse effects and interactions with other drugs. [NIH]

Phonophoresis: Use of ultrasound to increase the percutaneous adsorption of drugs. [NIH]

Phosphorus: A non-metallic element that is found in the blood, muscles, nevers, bones, and teeth, and is a component of adenosine triphosphate (ATP; the primary energy source for the body's cells.) [NIH]

Physical Therapy: The restoration of function and the prevention of disability following disease or injury with the use of light, heat, cold, water, electricity, ultrasound, and exercise. [NIH]

Physiologic: Having to do with the functions of the body. When used in the phrase "physiologic age," it refers to an age assigned by general health, as opposed to calendar age. [NIH]

Physiology: The science that deals with the life processes and functions of organismus, their cells, tissues, and organs. [NIH]

Pilot study: The initial study examining a new method or treatment. [NIH]

Plants: Multicellular, eukaryotic life forms of the kingdom Plantae. They are characterized by a mainly photosynthetic mode of nutrition; essentially unlimited growth at localized regions of cell divisions (meristems); cellulose within cells providing rigidity; the absence of organs of locomotion; absense of nervous and sensory systems; and an alteration of haploid and diploid generations. [NIH]

Plaque: A clear zone in a bacterial culture grown on an agar plate caused by localized destruction of bacterial cells by a bacteriophage. The concentration of infective virus in a fluid can be estimated by applying the fluid to a culture and counting the number of. [NIH]

Pneumonia: Inflammation of the lungs. [NIH]

Poisoning: A condition or physical state produced by the ingestion, injection or inhalation of, or exposure to a deleterious agent. [NIH]

Polyethylene: A vinyl polymer made from ethylene. It can be branched or linear. Branched or low-density polyethylene is tough and pliable but not to the same degree as linear polyethylene. Linear or high-density polyethylene has a greater hardness and tensile strength. Polyethylene is used in a variety of products, including implants and prostheses. [NIH]

Posterior: Situated in back of, or in the back part of, or affecting the back or dorsal surface of the body. In lower animals, it refers to the caudal end of the body. [EU]

Postoperative: After surgery. [NIH]

Post-traumatic: Occurring as a result of or after injury. [EU]

Potentiating: A degree of synergism which causes the exposure of the organism to a harmful substance to worsen a disease already contracted. [NIH]

Practice Guidelines: Directions or principles presenting current or future rules of policy for the health care practitioner to assist him in patient care decisions regarding diagnosis, therapy, or related clinical circumstances. The guidelines may be developed by government agencies at any level, institutions, professional societies, governing boards, or by the convening of expert panels. The guidelines form a basis for the evaluation of all aspects of health care and delivery. [NIH]

Precipitating Factors: Factors associated with the definitive onset of a disease, illness, accident, behavioral response, or course of action. Usually one factor is more important or more obviously recognizable than others, if several are involved, and one may often be regarded as "necessary". Examples include exposure to specific disease; amount or level of an infectious organism, drug, or noxious agent, etc. [NIH]

Precursor: Something that precedes. In biological processes, a substance from which another, usually more active or mature substance is formed. In clinical medicine, a sign or symptom that heralds another. [EU]

Predisposition: A latent susceptibility to disease which may be activated under certain conditions, as by stress. [EU]

Presynaptic: Situated proximal to a synapse, or occurring before the synapse is crossed. [EU]

Prevalence: The total number of cases of a given disease in a specified population at a designated time. It is differentiated from incidence, which refers to the number of new cases in the population at a given time. [NIH]

Probe: An instrument used in exploring cavities, or in the detection and dilatation of strictures, or in demonstrating the potency of channels; an elongated instrument for exploring or sounding body cavities. [NIH]

Progressive: Advancing; going forward; going from bad to worse; increasing in scope or severity. [EU]

Projection: A defense mechanism, operating unconsciously, whereby that which is emotionally unacceptable in the self is rejected and attributed (projected) to others. [NIH]

Prolactin: Pituitary lactogenic hormone. A polypeptide hormone with a molecular weight of about 23,000. It is essential in the induction of lactation in mammals at parturition and is synergistic with estrogen. The hormone also brings about the release of progesterone from lutein cells, which renders the uterine mucosa suited for the embedding of the ovum should fertilization occur. [NIH]

Prophase: The first phase of cell division, in which the chromosomes become visible, the nucleus starts to lose its identity, the spindle appears, and the centrioles migrate toward opposite poles. [NIH]

Propranolol: A widely used non-cardioselective beta-adrenergic antagonist. Propranolol is used in the treatment or prevention of many disorders including acute myocardial infarction, arrhythmias, angina pectoris, hypertension, hypertensive emergencies, hyperthyroidism, migraine, pheochromocytoma, menopause, and anxiety. [NIH]

Protein S: The vitamin K-dependent cofactor of activated protein C. Together with protein C, it inhibits the action of factors VIIIa and Va. A deficiency in protein S can lead to recurrent venous and arterial thrombosis. [NIH]

Proteins: Polymers of amino acids linked by peptide bonds. The specific sequence of amino acids determines the shape and function of the protein. [NIH]

Proteolytic: 1. Pertaining to, characterized by, or promoting proteolysis. 2. An enzyme that promotes proteolysis (= the splitting of proteins by hydrolysis of the peptide bonds with formation of smaller polypeptides). [EU]

Protocol: The detailed plan for a clinical trial that states the trial's rationale, purpose, drug or vaccine dosages, length of study, routes of administration, who may participate, and other aspects of trial design. [NIH]

Proximal: Nearest; closer to any point of reference; opposed to distal. [EU]

Pruritic: Pertaining to or characterized by pruritus. [EU]

Psoriasis: A common genetically determined, chronic, inflammatory skin disease characterized by rounded erythematous, dry, scaling patches. The lesions have a predilection for nails, scalp, genitalia, extensor surfaces, and the lumbosacral region. Accelerated epidermopoiesis is considered to be the fundamental pathologic feature in psoriasis. [NIH]

Psychic: Pertaining to the psyche or to the mind; mental. [EU]

Psychoactive: Those drugs which alter sensation, mood, consciousness or other psychological or behavioral functions. [NIH]

Psychogenesis: The origin and development of the psychic, however defined: of behavior, of mental or psychological processes, of mind, or of personality. [NIH]

Psychogenic: Produced or caused by psychic or mental factors rather than organic factors. [EU]

Psychological Techniques: Methods used in the diagnosis and treatment of behavioral, personality, and mental disorders. [NIH]

Psychosis: A mental disorder characterized by gross impairment in reality testing as evidenced by delusions, hallucinations, markedly incoherent speech, or disorganized and agitated behaviour without apparent awareness on the part of the patient of the incomprehensibility of his behaviour; the term is also used in a more general sense to refer to mental disorders in which mental functioning is sufficiently impaired as to interfere grossly with the patient's capacity to meet the ordinary demands of life. Historically, the term has been applied to many conditions, e.g. manic-depressive psychosis, that were first described in psychotic patients, although many patients with the disorder are not judged psychotic. [EU]

Psychosomatic: Pertaining to the mind-body relationship; having bodily symptoms of psychic, emotional, or mental origin; called also psychophysiologic. [EU]

Public Policy: A course or method of action selected, usually by a government, from among alternatives to guide and determine present and future decisions. [NIH]

Pulse: The rhythmical expansion and contraction of an artery produced by waves of pressure caused by the ejection of blood from the left ventricle of the heart as it contracts. [NIH]

Pyogenic: Producing pus; pyopoietic (= liquid inflammation product made up of cells and a thin fluid called liquor puris). [EU]

Quality of Life: A generic concept reflecting concern with the modification and enhancement of life attributes, e.g., physical, political, moral and social environment. [NIH]

Race: A population within a species which exhibits general similarities within itself, but is both discontinuous and distinct from other populations of that species, though not sufficiently so as to achieve the status of a taxon. [NIH]

Racemic: Optically inactive but resolvable in the way of all racemic compounds. [NIH]

Radiological: Pertaining to radiodiagnostic and radiotherapeutic procedures, and interventional radiology or other planning and guiding medical radiology. [NIH]

Radiopharmaceutical: Any medicinal product which, when ready for use, contains one or more radionuclides (radioactive isotopes) included for a medicinal purpose. [NIH]

Rage: Fury; violent, intense anger. [NIH]

Randomized: Describes an experiment or clinical trial in which animal or human subjects are assigned by chance to separate groups that compare different treatments. [NIH]

Receptor: A molecule inside or on the surface of a cell that binds to a specific substance and causes a specific physiologic effect in the cell. [NIH]

Receptors, Serotonin: Cell-surface proteins that bind serotonin and trigger intracellular changes which influence the behavior of cells. Several types of serotonin receptors have been recognized which differ in their pharmacology, molecular biology, and mode of action. [NIH]

Rectum: The last 8 to 10 inches of the large intestine. [NIH]

Refer: To send or direct for treatment, aid, information, de decision. [NIH]

Reflex: An involuntary movement or exercise of function in a part, excited in response to a stimulus applied to the periphery and transmitted to the brain or spinal cord. [NIH]

Refractory: Not readily yielding to treatment. [EU]

Regimen: A treatment plan that specifies the dosage, the schedule, and the duration of treatment. [NIH]

Regurgitation: A backward flowing, as the casting up of undigested food, or the backward flowing of blood into the heart, or between the chambers of the heart when a valve is incompetent. [EU]

Relaxant: 1. Lessening or reducing tension. 2. An agent that lessens tension. [EU]

Resorption: The loss of substance through physiologic or pathologic means, such as loss of dentin and cementum of a tooth, or of the alveolar process of the mandible or maxilla. [EU]

Respiration: The act of breathing with the lungs, consisting of inspiration, or the taking into the lungs of the ambient air, and of expiration, or the expelling of the modified air which contains more carbon dioxide than the air taken in (Blakiston's Gould Medical Dictionary, 4th ed.). This does not include tissue respiration (= oxygen consumption) or cell respiration (= cell respiration). [NIH]

Restless legs: Legs characterized by or showing inability to remain at rest. [EU]

Retrograde: 1. Moving backward or against the usual direction of flow. 2. Degenerating, deteriorating, or catabolic. [EU]

Retrospective: Looking back at events that have already taken place. [NIH]

Rheumatoid: Resembling rheumatism. [EU]

Rheumatoid arthritis: A form of arthritis, the cause of which is unknown, although infection, hypersensitivity, hormone imbalance and psychologic stress have been suggested as possible causes. [NIH]

Risk factor: A habit, trait, condition, or genetic alteration that increases a person's chance of developing a disease. [NIH]

Rod: A reception for vision, located in the retina. [NIH]

Saliva: The clear, viscous fluid secreted by the salivary glands and mucous glands of the mouth. It contains mucins, water, organic salts, and ptylin. [NIH]

Salivary: The duct that convey saliva to the mouth. [NIH]

Schizoid: Having qualities resembling those found in greater degree in schizophrenics; a person of schizoid personality. [NIH]

Schizophrenia: A mental disorder characterized by a special type of disintegration of the personality. [NIH]

Schizotypal Personality Disorder: A personality disorder in which there are oddities of thought (magical thinking, paranoid ideation, suspiciousness), perception (illusions, depersonalization), speech (digressive, vague, overelaborate), and behavior (inappropriate affect in social interactions, frequently social isolation) that are not severe enough to characterize schizophrenia. [NIH]

Sclerosis: A pathological process consisting of hardening or fibrosis of an anatomical structure, often a vessel or a nerve. [NIH]

Screening: Checking for disease when there are no symptoms. [NIH]

Secretion: 1. The process of elaborating a specific product as a result of the activity of a gland; this activity may range from separating a specific substance of the blood to the elaboration of a new chemical substance. 2. Any substance produced by secretion. [EU]

Sedative: 1. Allaying activity and excitement. 2. An agent that allays excitement. [EU]

Seizures: Clinical or subclinical disturbances of cortical function due to a sudden, abnormal, excessive, and disorganized discharge of brain cells. Clinical manifestations include abnormal motor, sensory and psychic phenomena. Recurrent seizures are usually referred to as epilepsy or "seizure disorder." [NIH]

Semicircular canal: Three long canals of the bony labyrinth of the ear, forming loops and opening into the vestibule by five openings. [NIH]

Semisynthetic: Produced by chemical manipulation of naturally occurring substances. [EU]

Sensor: A device designed to respond to physical stimuli such as temperature, light, magnetism or movement and transmit resulting impulses for interpretation, recording, movement, or operating control. [NIH]

Septicaemia: A term originally used to denote a putrefactive process in the body, but now usually referring to infection with pyogenic micro-organisms; a genus of Diptera; the severe type of infection in which the blood stream is invaded by large numbers of the causal. [NIH]

Sequela: Any lesion or affection following or caused by an attack of disease. [EU]

Serotonin: A biochemical messenger and regulator, synthesized from the essential amino acid L-tryptophan. In humans it is found primarily in the central nervous system, gastrointestinal tract, and blood platelets. Serotonin mediates several important physiological functions including neurotransmission, gastrointestinal motility, hemostasis, and cardiovascular integrity. Multiple receptor families (receptors, serotonin) explain the broad physiological actions and distribution of this biochemical mediator. [NIH]

Serum: The clear liquid part of the blood that remains after blood cells and clotting proteins have been removed. [NIH]

Shock: The general bodily disturbance following a severe injury; an emotional or moral upset occasioned by some disturbing or unexpected experience; disruption of the circulation, which can upset all body functions: sometimes referred to as circulatory shock. [NIH]

Side effect: A consequence other than the one(s) for which an agent or measure is used, as the adverse effects produced by a drug, especially on a tissue or organ system other than the one sought to be benefited by its administration. [EU]

Signs and Symptoms: Clinical manifestations that can be either objective when observed by a physician, or subjective when perceived by the patient. [NIH]

Skeletal: Having to do with the skeleton (boney part of the body). [NIH]

Skeleton: The framework that supports the soft tissues of vertebrate animals and protects many of their internal organs. The skeletons of vertebrates are made of bone and/or cartilage. [NIH]

Skull: The skeleton of the head including the bones of the face and the bones enclosing the brain. [NIH]

Sleep apnea: A serious, potentially life-threatening breathing disorder characterized by repeated cessation of breathing due to either collapse of the upper airway during sleep or absence of respiratory effort. [NIH]

Sleep Bruxism: A sleep disorder characterized by grinding and clenching of the teeth and forceful lateral or protrusive jaw movements. Sleep bruxism may be associated with tooth injuries; temporomandibular joint disorders; sleep disturbances; and other conditions. [NIH]

Sleep Stages: Periods of sleep manifested by changes in EEG activity and certain behavioral correlates; includes Stage 1: sleep onset, drowsy sleep; Stage 2: light sleep; Stages 3 and 4: delta sleep, light sleep, deep sleep, telencephalic sleep. [NIH]

Smooth muscle: Muscle that performs automatic tasks, such as constricting blood vessels. [NIH]

Snoring: Rough, noisy breathing during sleep, due to vibration of the uvula and soft palate. [NIH]

Social Environment: The aggregate of social and cultural institutions, forms, patterns, and processes that influence the life of an individual or community. [NIH]

Soft tissue: Refers to muscle, fat, fibrous tissue, blood vessels, or other supporting tissue of the body. [NIH]

Sound wave: An alteration of properties of an elastic medium, such as pressure, particle displacement, or density, that propagates through the medium, or a superposition of such alterations. [NIH]

Spasm: An involuntary contraction of a muscle or group of muscles. Spasms may involve skeletal muscle or smooth muscle. [NIH]

Spasmodic: Of the nature of a spasm. [EU]

Specialist: In medicine, one who concentrates on 1 special branch of medical science. [NIH]

Species: A taxonomic category subordinate to a genus (or subgenus) and superior to a subspecies or variety, composed of individuals possessing common characters distinguishing them from other categories of individuals of the same taxonomic level. In taxonomic nomenclature, species are designated by the genus name followed by a Latin or Latinized adjective or noun. [EU]

Spinal cord: The main trunk or bundle of nerves running down the spine through holes in the spinal bone (the vertebrae) from the brain to the level of the lower back. [NIH]

Splint: A rigid appliance used for the immobilization of a part or for the correction of deformity. [NIH]

Stabilization: The creation of a stable state. [EU]

Standardize: To compare with or conform to a standard; to establish standards. [EU]

Steel: A tough, malleable, iron-based alloy containing up to, but no more than, two percent carbon and often other metals. It is used in medicine and dentistry in implants and instrumentation. [NIH]

Stimulus: That which can elicit or evoke action (response) in a muscle, nerve, gland or other excitable issue, or cause an augmenting action upon any function or metabolic process. [NIH]

Stomach: An organ of digestion situated in the left upper quadrant of the abdomen between the termination of the esophagus and the beginning of the duodenum. [NIH]

Stomatitis: Inflammation of the oral mucosa, due to local or systemic factors which may involve the buccal and labial mucosa, palate, tongue, floor of the mouth, and the gingivae. [EU]

Stomatognathic System: The mouth, teeth, jaws, pharynx, and related structures as they relate to mastication, deglutition, and speech. [NIH]

Stress: Forcibly exerted influence; pressure. Any condition or situation that causes strain or tension. Stress may be either physical or psychologic, or both. [NIH]

Subacute: Somewhat acute; between acute and chronic. [EU]

Subarachnoid: Situated or occurring between the arachnoid and the pia mater. [EU]

Subclinical: Without clinical manifestations; said of the early stage(s) of an infection or other disease or abnormality before symptoms and signs become apparent or detectable by clinical examination or laboratory tests, or of a very mild form of an infection or other disease or abnormality. [EU]

Substrate: A substance upon which an enzyme acts. [EU]

Supplementation: Adding nutrients to the diet. [NIH]

Suppression: A conscious exclusion of disapproved desire contrary with repression, in which the process of exclusion is not conscious. [NIH]

Symptomatic: Having to do with symptoms, which are signs of a condition or disease. [NIH]

Symptomatic treatment: Therapy that eases symptoms without addressing the cause of disease. [NIH]

Symptomatology: 1. That branch of medicine with treats of symptoms; the systematic discussion of symptoms. 2. The combined symptoms of a disease. [EU]

Synapse: The region where the processes of two neurons come into close contiguity, and the nervous impulse passes from one to the other; the fibers of the two are intermeshed, but, according to the general view, there is no direct contiguity. [NIH]

Synapsis: The pairing between homologous chromosomes of maternal and paternal origin during the prophase of meiosis, leading to the formation of gametes. [NIH]

Synaptic: Pertaining to or affecting a synapse (= site of functional apposition between neurons, at which an impulse is transmitted from one neuron to another by electrical or chemical means); pertaining to synapsis (= pairing off in point-for-point association of homologous chromosomes from the male and female pronuclei during the early prophase of meiosis). [EU]

Synergistic: Acting together; enhancing the effect of another force or agent. [EU]

Systemic: Affecting the entire body. [NIH]

Tardive: Marked by lateness, late; said of a disease in which the characteristic lesion is late in appearing. [EU]

Telencephalon: Paired anteriolateral evaginations of the prosencephalon plus the lamina terminalis. The cerebral hemispheres are derived from it. Many authors consider cerebrum a synonymous term to telencephalon, though a minority include diencephalon as part of the cerebrum (Anthoney, 1994). [NIH]

Temporal: One of the two irregular bones forming part of the lateral surfaces and base of the skull, and containing the organs of hearing. [NIH]

Temporal Muscle: A masticatory muscle whose action is closing the jaws; its posterior portion retracts the mandible. [NIH]

Temporomandibular Joint Dysfunction Syndrome: A symptom complex consisting of pain, muscle tenderness, clicking in the joint, and limitation or alteration of mandibular movement. The symptoms are subjective and manifested primarily in the masticatory muscles rather than the temporomandibular joint itself. Etiologic factors are uncertain but include occlusal dysharmony and psychophysiologic factors. [NIH]

Tendon: A discrete band of connective tissue mainly composed of parallel bundles of collagenous fibers by which muscles are attached, or two muscles bellies joined. [NIH]

Therapeutics: The branch of medicine which is concerned with the treatment of diseases, palliative or curative. [NIH]

Thermal: Pertaining to or characterized by heat. [EU]

Third Ventricle: A narrow cleft inferior to the corpus callosum, within the diencephalon, between the paired thalami. Its floor is formed by the hypothalamus, its anterior wall by the lamina terminalis, and its roof by ependyma. It communicates with the fourth ventricle by the cerebral aqueduct, and with the lateral ventricles by the interventricular foramina. [NIH]

Threshold: For a specified sensory modality (e. g. light, sound, vibration), the lowest level (absolute threshold) or smallest difference (difference threshold, difference limen) or intensity of the stimulus discernible in prescribed conditions of stimulation. [NIH]

Thrush: A disease due to infection with species of fungi of the genus Candida. [NIH]

Thyroid: A gland located near the windpipe (trachea) that produces thyroid hormone, which helps regulate growth and metabolism. [NIH]

Tic: An involuntary compulsive, repetitive, stereotyped movement, resembling a purposeful movement because it is coordinated and involves muscles in their normal synergistic relationships; tics usually involve the face and shoulders. [EU]

Tissue: A group or layer of cells that are alike in type and work together to perform a specific function. [NIH]

Tomography: Imaging methods that result in sharp images of objects located on a chosen plane and blurred images located above or below the plane. [NIH]

Tone: 1. The normal degree of vigour and tension; in muscle, the resistance to passive elongation or stretch; tonus. 2. A particular quality of sound or of voice. 3. To make permanent, or to change, the colour of silver stain by chemical treatment, usually with a heavy metal. [EU]

Tonicity: The normal state of muscular tension. [NIH]

Tonus: A state of slight tension usually present in muscles even when they are not undergoing active contraction. [NIH]

Tooth Injuries: Traumatic or other damage to teeth including fractures (tooth fractures) or displacements (tooth luxation). [NIH]

Tooth Loss: The failure to retain teeth as a result of disease or injury. [NIH]

Tooth Socket: A hollow part of the alveolar process of the maxilla or mandible where each tooth fits and is attached via the peridontal ligament. [NIH]

Topical: On the surface of the body. [NIH]

Toxic: Having to do with poison or something harmful to the body. Toxic substances usually cause unwanted side effects. [NIH]

Toxicity: The quality of being poisonous, especially the degree of virulence of a toxic microbe or of a poison. [EU]

Toxicology: The science concerned with the detection, chemical composition, and pharmacologic action of toxic substances or poisons and the treatment and prevention of toxic manifestations. [NIH]

Toxin: A poison; frequently used to refer specifically to a protein produced by some higher plants, certain animals, and pathogenic bacteria, which is highly toxic for other living organisms. Such substances are differentiated from the simple chemical poisons and the vegetable alkaloids by their high molecular weight and antigenicity. [EU]

Trachea: The cartilaginous and membranous tube descending from the larynx and branching into the right and left main bronchi. [NIH]

Traction: The act of pulling. [NIH]

Transcutaneous: Transdermal. [EU]

Transcutaneous Electric Nerve Stimulation: Electrical stimulation of nerves and/or muscles to relieve pain; it is used less frequently to produce anesthesia. The optimal placements of electrodes or "trigger points" may correspond with acupuncture analgesia points. TENS is sometimes referred to as acupuncture-like when using a low frequency stimulus. [NIH]

Transfection: The uptake of naked or purified DNA into cells, usually eukaryotic. It is analogous to bacterial transformation. [NIH]

Transmitter: A chemical substance which effects the passage of nerve impulses from one cell to the other at the synapse. [NIH]

Trauma: Any injury, wound, or shock, must frequently physical or structural shock, producing a disturbance. [NIH]

Tremor: Cyclical movement of a body part that can represent either a physiologic process or a manifestation of disease. Intention or action tremor, a common manifestation of cerebellar diseases, is aggravated by movement. In contrast, resting tremor is maximal when there is no attempt at voluntary movement, and occurs as a relatively frequent manifestation of Parkinson disease. [NIH]

Trigeminal: Cranial nerve V. It is sensory for the eyeball, the conjunctiva, the eyebrow, the skin of face and scalp, the teeth, the mucous membranes in the mouth and nose, and is motor to the muscles of mastication. [NIH]

Trigeminal Ganglion: The semilunar-shaped ganglion containing the cells of origin of most of the sensory fibers of the trigeminal nerve. It is situated within the dural cleft on the cerebral surface of the petrous portion of the temporal bone and gives off the ophthalmic, maxillary, and part of the mandibular nerves. [NIH]

Trigeminal Nerve: The 5th and largest cranial nerve. The trigeminal nerve is a mixed motor and sensory nerve. The larger sensory part forms the ophthalmic, mandibular, and maxillary nerves which carry afferents sensitive to external or internal stimuli from the skin, muscles, and joints of the face and mouth and from the teeth. Most of these fibers originate from cells of the trigeminal ganglion and project to the trigeminal nucleus of the brain stem. The smaller motor part arises from the brain stem trigeminal motor nucleus and innervates the muscles of mastication. [NIH]

Trigeminal Nuclei: Nuclei of the trigeminal nerve situated in the brain stem. They include the nucleus of the spinal trigeminal tract (spinal trigeminal nucleus), the principal sensory nucleus, the mesencephalic nucleus, and the motor nucleus. [NIH]

Trigger zone: Dolorogenic zone (= producing or causing pain). [EU]

Tryptophan: An essential amino acid that is necessary for normal growth in infants and for nitrogen balance in adults. It is a precursor serotonin and niacin. [NIH]

Tumour: 1. Swelling, one of the cardinal signs of inflammations; morbid enlargement. 2. A new growth of tissue in which the multiplication of cells is uncontrolled and progressive; called also neoplasm. [EU]

Turbinates: The scroll-like bony plates with curved margins on the lateral wall of the nasal cavity. [NIH]

Unconscious: Experience which was once conscious, but was subsequently rejected, as the "personal unconscious". [NIH]

Uterus: The small, hollow, pear-shaped organ in a woman's pelvis. This is the organ in which a fetus develops. Also called the womb. [NIH]

Uvula: Uvula palatinae; specifically, the tongue-like process which projects from the middle of the posterior edge of the soft palate. [NIH]

Vaccine: A substance or group of substances meant to cause the immune system to respond to a tumor or to microorganisms, such as bacteria or viruses. [NIH]

Vagina: The muscular canal extending from the uterus to the exterior of the body. Also called the birth canal. [NIH]

Vaginitis: Inflammation of the vagina characterized by pain and a purulent discharge. [NIH]

Vascular: Pertaining to blood vessels or indicative of a copious blood supply. [EU]

Vein: Vessel-carrying blood from various parts of the body to the heart. [NIH]

Venlafaxine: An antidepressant drug that is being evaluated for the treatment of hot flashes in women who have breast cancer. [NIH]

Ventricle: One of the two pumping chambers of the heart. The right ventricle receives oxygen-poor blood from the right atrium and pumps it to the lungs through the pulmonary artery. The left ventricle receives oxygen-rich blood from the left atrium and pumps it to the body through the aorta. [NIH]

Vertebrae: A bony unit of the segmented spinal column. [NIH]

Vertigo: An illusion of movement; a sensation as if the external world were revolving around the patient (objective vertigo) or as if he himself were revolving in space (subjective vertigo). The term is sometimes erroneously used to mean any form of dizziness. [EU]

Vestibule: A small, oval, bony chamber of the labyrinth. The vestibule contains the utricle and saccule, organs which are part of the balancing apparatus of the ear. [NIH]

Veterinary Medicine: The medical science concerned with the prevention, diagnosis, and treatment of diseases in animals. [NIH]

Virus: Submicroscopic organism that causes infectious disease. In cancer therapy, some viruses may be made into vaccines that help the body build an immune response to, and kill, tumor cells. [NIH]

Vivo: Outside of or removed from the body of a living organism. [NIH]

Volition: Voluntary activity without external compulsion. [NIH]

Windpipe: A rigid tube, 10 cm long, extending from the cricoid cartilage to the upper border of the fifth thoracic vertebra. [NIH]

Withdrawal: 1. A pathological retreat from interpersonal contact and social involvement, as may occur in schizophrenia, depression, or schizoid avoidant and schizotypal personality disorders. 2. (DSM III-R) A substance-specific organic brain syndrome that follows the cessation of use or reduction in intake of a psychoactive substance that had been regularly used to induce a state of intoxication. [EU]

X-ray: High-energy radiation used in low doses to diagnose diseases and in high doses to treat cancer. [NIH]

INDEX

Printed in the United States
117876LV00006B/218/A